W9-AUI-205

The public's awareness and knowledge about stroke lags far behind that of heart disease and cancer. This is partly explained by the complexity of brain function and the many varied symptoms and presentations of stroke. Williams' *Stroke Diaries* is clearly aimed at stroke patients and their families and loved ones and at the public in general. He skillfully tries to narrow the information gap by using the stories of real stroke patients.

Life is a series of stories. In wonderful, very readable prose, Williams recounts his patients' stories. Many of the patients are true victims of poverty, circumstances, and their own weaknesses. Despite this they often show bravery and heroism in battling the disabilities that remain after their strokes. Williams uses each stroke patient's story as a springboard to deliver important background information about stroke—its symptoms, causes, diagnosis, and treatment. Necessarily this involves some understanding about the brain—what it looks like, how it works, how strokes cause injury. The book is peppered with simple diagrams, pictures, and tables that help skillfully to convey the information.

Williams' prose is simple but elegant and a pleasure to read. I heartily recommend this book to everyone who seeks information about all of the facets of stroke.

—Louis R. Caplan, MD, Professor of Neurology, Harvard Medical School, Boston, MA

Stroke Diaries offers vivid, informative and at times heart-wrenching stories about stroke survivors, and in the process emphasizes the importance of educating everyone about the warning signs and symptoms of stroke, a condition that affects nearly 800,000 Americans each year and is the third leading cause of death in the United States. Dr. Williams combines lucid writing with practical, take-home information about stroke that should inform stroke patients, their families, and the public at large.

—Timothy A. Pedley, MD, Henry and Lucy Moses Professor of Neurology, Chairman, Department of Neurology, Neurologist-in-Chief, The Neurological Institute of New York, Columbia University Medical Center, New York, NY

Stroke is the third most common cause of death, affecting 780,000 people each year, with a cumulative number of survivors coming to six million. The toll on individuals, families, and society makes the problem an urgent one to solve. After a stroke, depression compounds the physical injury and debility. An effective treatment, tissue plasminogen activator (tPA), is available but is used in only 3% of all cases. A public education program is sorely needed and the void is filled by this spirited book.

The author, Olajide Williams, a Columbia University neurologist, has mounted the program at Harlem Hospital in New York City. He illustrates all aspects of stroke epidemiology and pathophysiology in poignant case histories from his own files, stories told in a way that makes each one human. In a deprived population, adult education is a challenge, so Dr. Williams has gone to grade schools, teaching children how to recognize stroke and how to get the adult patients to the hospital.

The book is written in a lively and clear fashion. 17 chapters cover epidemiology, symptoms, stroke prevention, emergency treatment and certified stroke centers, hemine-glect, locked-in syndrome, man-in-a-barrel, sex and psychosocial aspects, and recovery from stroke. The large intended audience of survivors and their families is no longer neglected.

—Lewis P. Rowland, MD, The Neurological Institute of New York, Columbia University Medical Center, New York, NY

STROKE DIARIES

*A Guide for Survivors
and Their Families*

OLAJIDE WILLIAMS, MD, MS

Department of Neurology
Columbia University Medical Center
Neurological Institute of New York
Harlem Hospital Center
New York, NY

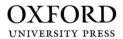

2010

OXFORD
UNIVERSITY PRESS

Oxford University Press, Inc., publishes works that further
Oxford University's objective of excellence
in research, scholarship, and education.

Oxford   New York
Auckland   Cape Town   Dar es Salaam   Hong Kong   Karachi
Kuala Lumpur   Madrid   Melbourne   Mexico City   Nairobi
New Delhi   Shanghai   Taipei   Toronto

With offices in
Argentina   Austria   Brazil   Chile   Czech Republic   France   Greece
Guatemala   Hungary   Italy   Japan   Poland   Portugal   Singapore
South Korea   Switzerland   Thailand   Turkey   Ukraine   Vietnam

Published by Oxford University Press, Inc.
198 Madison Avenue, New York, New York 10016

www.oup.com

Oxford is a registered trademark of Oxford University Press

Library of Congress Cataloging-in-Publication Data
Williams, Olajide.
Stroke diaries : a guide for survivors and their families / Olajide Williams.
p.   cm.
Includes bibliographical references and index.
ISBN 978-0-19-974026-0
1. Cerebrovascular disease—Patients.
2. Cerebrovascular disease—Patients—Rehabilitation.   I. Title.
RC388.5.W475 2010
616.8′1—dc22
2009040075

1 3 5 7 9 8 6 4 2

Printed in the United States of America
on acid-free paper

I dedicate this book to Gloria Bynoe-Thomas, my muse...
Rest in Peace.

FOREWORD

Stroke continues to touch so many of our lives. Everyone probably has known someone who has had a stroke. Every 3 minutes someone dies of a stroke, and every 45 seconds someone has a stroke in the United States. Although stroke remains the third leading cause of death in the United States and the leading cause of serious disability, it continues to be underrecognized by the public. Too many people do not recognize the warning signs and fail to get the urgent treatments that can make a major difference in the quality of life after stroke. In the last 15 years, we have made major strides in our approach to acute stroke treatments. We have also learned much more about the many ways to prevent stroke. Stroke centers continue to be certified, and we are training more health care professionals to care for stroke. Yet, we still have so much more to do.

Dr. Olajide Williams has done a terrific job in helping paint the many portraits of stroke in his book, *Stroke Diaries*. I had the pleasure of knowing and working with Dr. Williams when he was a neurology resident at Columbia University. As a faculty member, I also watched him make major strides in improving the care of stroke patients at Harlem Hospital Center and create innovative public awareness campaigns about stroke. His energy, enthusiasm, and passion are always evident, and he continues to make a real difference.

This book is another way that Dr. Williams has continued his crusade to reduce stroke. His colorful, heart-wrenching stories of patients and families who have experienced stroke serve to illustrate the many issues surrounding this important medical problem. He uses these as a springboard to provide helpful facts about the prevention, diagnosis, treatment, and recovery of stroke. Whether you are a stroke survivor, a family member, or a person at risk, there are helpful facts in this book for everyone. We need more books like this to spread the word about stroke. I hope each person who learns something from reading this book will help tell others some useful stroke facts and reduce the impact of stroke on our loved ones.

Ralph L. Sacco, MD, MS, FAHA, FAAN
Olemberg Family Chair in Neurological Disorders and
Chairman of Neurology
Neurologist-in-Chief, Jackson Memorial Hospital
Miller Professor of Neurology, Epidemiology, and Human Genetics
University of Miami, FL

PREFACE

Carried by a wind of voices—voices of strangers on hospital beds—I arrived at a decision point. To write or not to write? I have never written a book before. Scholarly articles—yes. Book chapters in major medical texts—yes. But a departure from the rules—a book from the heart about patients I have treated—this was a risk I was not prepared to take, one that I felt ill equipped to attempt. But the voices grew louder, silent cries from sick souls: a man who could not speak, a woman who could not see, a man who could not move, and so many more.

I can no longer suppress their stories.

So I have freed myself, allowed my heart to speak out, to dictate the pace and direction of its freedom, to give voices to heroes—stroke heroes—voices from whom I hope we can all learn.

ACKNOWLEDGMENTS

To my wife, Buki, thank you for your support and sacrifice without which this book would not have been possible. To my children, Lola and Tobi, you are my all-in-all. My sister, Olatoun, you are the fury behind this book: I carry your passion—remember the abyss of will. My parents, Dr Gabi Williams and Mrs Abisola Williams, you are the foundation of my stability. My sister Mope and my brother Tunde, you live in the center of my heart. My cousin Remi Oshikanlu and good friends Doug E Fresh and Andreas Williams, thank you for encouraging me to keep writing until the very end.

I must also thank Dr. John Brust, my incredible mentor and friend, for his editorial eye. Dr. Lewis Rowland, Hazella Rollins-LaVar, Dr. Daniel Labovitz, Dr. Ralph Sacco, and Dr. Mehmet Oz, thank you all for reviewing my manuscript and making helpful comments. To Rochelle DeOlivera, speech pathologist, thank you for your help with speech and swallowing information. To Maiken Jacobs, occupational therapist: You are special. I cannot imagine what I would have done without you! Thank you for always bringing out the best in me, one chapter at a time. To Thom Graves of Thom Graves Media, thank you for turning my vision into wonderful illustrations. To my editor at Oxford University Press, Craig Panner, thank you for believing in this book long before it was accepted for publication, and for making key suggestions that greatly enhanced my original manuscript.

Finally, to all my patients—the source of my inspiration—I thank you for teaching me so much about life in its purest form. I will always be at your service.

We all have different views of stroke. For some, it is a view of a loved one or close friend who has suffered a stroke; for others, it is a view of strangers with awkward steps or crooked smiles; for others still, it is an empty view—an invisible world filled with afflicted people they would rather not see; and for me, it is a view of signs and symptoms, different treatments and prescriptions, and countless patients who are dead and alive. Yet none of these views are enough: they are not enough to see the panoramic struggle for hope inside a stroke patient's mind or watch the drama of depression unfold. These views are all insufficient, obscured by different angles, different points of view. We need to recognize all of stroke's faces wherever it appears: inside emergency rooms, on our city streets and rural roads, in our backyards, and inside our homes. We need a holistic view of stroke.

Anosodiaphoria is a term used to describe a patient's indifference or inability to experience an emotional reaction to his or her paralyzing symptoms of stroke. And while it is hard to imagine such a syndrome, it is harder to accept the anosodiaphoria that shrouds our public health efforts against stroke. For too long we have seen stroke's footprints without hearing its footsteps: footsteps that stalk our alleys like a thief in the night, mugging brain cells of unsuspecting victims every 45 seconds, and stealing a life every 3 minutes.

Why is the number one cause of adult disability invisible? Why are still only approximately 3% of stroke patients in the United States treated emergently with a drug that works, that can potentially reverse disability, and that has been around for more than a decade? (In some countries like the United Kingdom, this number is less than 1%.) Why is the crisis of stroke such a public health mystery?

With more than 780,000 strokes occurring every year in America, the equivalent of almost 10 New York Giants football stadiums, it is clear that stroke awareness needs a transformation. Six million stroke survivors in this country alone deserve it; and while one transforming act stands out in my mind, there are innumerable such acts touching four out of every five American households.

On December 31, 2005, Dick Clark, American bandstand's sweetheart, startled the world. He appeared on television for his traditional New Year's Eve celebration and countdown. This was the first time America had seen him since his stroke—his crooked smile and paralyzed limb; it was the first time they heard his slurred words, which tumbled over one another as the crystal ball fell from the sky.

As a spokesperson for the National Stroke Association, I was invited to appear on Fox News' Bill O'Reilly show and NBC's Access Hollywood. They wanted me to weigh in on the public discourse surrounding his appearance and provide an expert opinion about his stroke. According to some media pundits, Dick Clark's appearance made millions of Americans uncomfortable on what should have been a festive night. They said his disability was disconcerting, and that the network should not have sanctioned his appearance in that condition.

I disagreed.

To me, Dick Clark showed great courage that night. He was a flag bearer, using his platform to promote awareness—just by showing up and sending a subliminal message to engage our higher selves.

Words can make worlds inside our imagination—they can create powerful illusions, but they cannot replace the aesthetic experience of real life. No matter how dramatic the description or how inspiring the prose, words cannot reproduce the ravages of stroke in a person's life. I say this because I am not qualified to attempt this feat; I only wish to share stories told from my humble perspective.

It is true that knowledge is power, but knowledge without motivation is powerless. This book strives to weave these basic truths together through a series of human stories and commentaries. It is an attempt to humanize stroke: to dispel the myths and reveal unashamed truth. It is my personal stroke diary: a collection of clinical experiences, each of which was inspired by a real patient. The characters have been altered, and several aspects of each episode have been fictionalized to protect the identity of patients and families. The episodes highlight stroke syndromes or complications, and the commentaries discuss their causes, prevention, and treatment or unique challenges across the continuum of stroke care.

The risk of recurrent stroke is high in those who have already had a stroke, and the risk of a first stroke may be higher in first-degree relatives of stroke survivors. This book was written in honor of stroke survivors, for them and for their families, although the general public may also benefit from its content.

Too often our professional guard dampens the personal touch we doctors hope to display. We hold back. We focus on the biological event and not the human event—on disease and not illness. Unknowingly, we sometimes stifle our ability to meaningfully connect with our patients and their loved ones. The result can be catastrophic: hopelessness, caregiver anxiety, and dangerous misconceptions about stroke.

Beyond the open windows of my clinic, I see a woman clothed in white, hovering in mid-air. There is no flaw in her. She is blindfolded, holding a set of scales, which are balanced at each end by ancient tonics labeled healing and cure. Her name is Themis—the ancient goddess of justice. After several minutes of watching her, her blindfolds fall off. Her eyes are like crystals, reflecting the golden-yellow sunset in the sky, and my shadow standing against the windowpane. When she looks straight at me, my thoughts become suspended in time. She asks me if I know the difference between healing and cure. She shows me the pain in my own heart, which still aches, despite my physical cure. And when I look closer at the balanced scales in her hands, I notice that the tonic labeled cure is filled with pills, and the one labeled healing is filled with kindness. An image then flashes in my mind. I see myself standing before a white wall upon which are hung all kinds of diplomas. I am holding tilted scales in my hands, at each end of which stand the tonics of healing and cure, and there is a black stethoscope around my neck. That was when I understood what all this meant: "Occasionally I will cure, often I can heal, but always I must care."

CONTENTS

STROKE
DIARIES

PART ONE

Causes, Prevention, and Emergency Treatment of Stroke

The Stroke that Came between Them

One of Anna's legs had been amputated above the knee due to complications from diabetes. It was replaced by a phantom limb, which doled out pain from imaginary joints every single day. And yet, Anna never cried—she never retreated. Instead, she looked forward, gazing towards infinity through a lens of hope, believing that tomorrow would bring healing.

Anna's husband disappeared a few days after her daughter was born. She came home one evening and he was gone—vanished without a trace: no note, no warnings, just empty closets and missing suitcases. Anna had no siblings, and no living parents—just two children, one of whom recently died. Her daughter, now 9 years old, suffered brain damage from the car accident that took her son's life. The young girl, like her mother, also suffered from diabetes and depended on Anna for her daily insulin shots. Anna did not have much money, but she had just enough to make her ineligible for government-assisted health insurance. She often relied on food stamps to feed her family, and emergency departments to refill her prescription drugs. The only luxury in Anna's life had been her dreams, but even these were gone—the death of her son caused a cut so deep that her hopes and dreams had bled out of her soul. Anna could still see her son's face. She could see it in her daughter's eyes. It was as though the accident occurred yesterday—she could still see the broken glass in the back seat of the car, and she could still hear herself screaming.

Some people arrange love in sequences such as, first love or second love, as though they are mountain peaks in our hearts separated by space and time. Others divide love into component parts like the ancient Greeks who had four words to describe love: "*eros*" for romantic love, "*storge*" for affection, "*philia*" for brotherly love, and "*agape*" for unconditional love. It has been said that agape best describes a mother's love for her child. They say that this form of love is the greatest love of all, and that it causes the greatest pain when it is lost. It is the only form of love that transcends self-preservation—the first law of nature, by lifting up the metaphysical truth that we are one people, and that sacrifice should not be for self, but for the greater unity of life. When Anna lost her son, aborted dreams of his future were replaced by pathological obsession over her daughter's health to the detriment of her own. Anna had started smoking cigarettes again—about one pack a day. She no longer went to emergency departments to refill her own prescriptions—she could not make time, and she often skipped meals or binged on junk food. Through her daughter's life, Anna breathed and moved, roaming through the routines of duty, and filled by the greatest pain.

When Anna woke up, a fugue by Bach was playing on her alarm clock radio: alternate-side parking had been suspended due to the recent snowstorm. When she opened her eyes, all she could see was pitch black, as though she were blind. When she tried to call her daughter in the next room, her words seemed stuck in her throat. Seized by fear, Anna called out once more with all of her might, but only silence streamed forth from the back of her mouth. Upon trying to climb out of bed, Anna fell onto the cold floor, which was where she lay for several hours until her daughter limped through the door.

It was the sound of the young child screaming that alarmed her neighbors that morning. The 9-year-old girl cried all day and all night, as she lay on the floor next to her mother, who could not speak and lacked the strength to get up. All Anna could do was look at her child with teary eyes, helpless and hopeless, and desperate on her bedroom floor.

Eventually, after much hesitation, her neighbors called the police. Anna would never harm her child, this her neighbors believed, but they feared the worst when they heard the young girl's cries and no one came to answer the front door.

It was as though Anna's body had struck a deal with a silent killer—one that slowly destroys internal organs without external signs. When she arrived at the hospital, Anna's blood pressure was dangerously high, and there were longstanding signs of internal organ damage, evidenced by her enlarged heart and tortuous blood vessels in the back of her eyes. And yet, prior to her stroke, her body did not reveal any telltale signs that her blood pressure was high.

I met Anna on the stroke unit 2 days later. She had dark blue eyes that were filled with fear. She looked older than her documented age, and a little unkempt. A long scar, which traversed facial contortions, was a remnant of the car accident. A stump leg further diminished her petite frame as she lay on the hospital bed, struggling in vain to speak and unable to move her good leg. She was becoming increasingly agitated as she tried painstakingly to tell me something of grave importance to her. But I could not understand her. My neurological examination on Anna revealed an unusual constellation of findings: her language skills were crippled by a debilitating difficulty with word production and sporadic defects in speech comprehension—a communication handicap called "aphasia." She was half blind and could no longer read through her working visual field. Remarkably, however, she could write, albeit strangely. I recognized the words "insulin" and "help me," but I could not make out the whole sentence, and Anna could not read what she wrote down. The stroke she suffered had caused a disconnection in her brain. It destroyed the bridge, which carried critical information from the right-brain to the left-brain, and it claimed her good leg.

After hours of intensity, I finally figured out what Anna was telling me: "My daughter needs insulin" she kept trying to say.

When I repeated what Anna was trying to tell me correctly back to her, tears began to fall from her eyes. Out of her watered eyes, more tears poured out like a deluge. Her cry was so loud that it made me tremble at her bedside, and then stumble over my own words as I tried to console her. And when her tears receded, I told Anna that I would make sure her daughter received her insulin. But there was something else I had to tell her: something far worse than the stroke itself. I knew about her son and the way he had died, which made it harder for me to begin these words:

"The social worker has been unable to find anyone to care for your daughter," I said, "Arrangements are being made to place her in a state-run foster home."

Comment

Stroke is not a terminal illness: it does not grow over time or spread to distant sites. Stroke can be cured or its effects curtailed. The word "stroke" is ubiquitous but often misunderstood. Contrary to popular opinion, stress is not the major cause of stroke. Indeed, the relationship between stress and stroke is complex and often indirect. Moreover, a stroke is not a heart attack; it does not occur in the heart, although having a heart attack puts one at risk for a stroke, and having a stroke puts one at risk for a heart attack. Stroke is a brain attack: a sudden brain catastrophe resulting from disease affecting the brain's blood vessels, which results in the death of brain tissue. These strokes ambush up to 780,000 Americans every year and cause 150,000 deaths each year in the United States. They are the leading cause of disability in adults and the third leading cause of death in America. Yet, most Americans do not know that stroke kills twice as many women as breast cancer every year.

There are two major types of stroke: a "dry" stroke, which is otherwise known as an "ischemic" stroke, and a "wet" stroke, which is otherwise known as a "hemorrhagic" stroke. The more common dry strokes, the type that afflicted Anna, are responsible for 80% of all strokes, and are caused by "lack of blood" to a given area of the brain due to downstream blockage of a blood vessel, usually by a blood clot (Fig. 1).

Affected blood vessels are usually riddled with a disease that hardens their walls, called atherosclerosis—a condition that is caused by smoking, and certain medical conditions, such as high blood pressure (the pressure in your arteries when your heart beats) and diabetes (high glucose levels in the blood)—both of which Anna had. However, offending blood clots may also occlude healthy-appearing blood vessels, especially in younger victims. The resulting deprivation of nourishment and oxygen delivery to specific regions of the brain leads to the death of almost two million brain cells every minute (unless the process is reversed), which manifests as symptoms of stroke: in Anna's case, aphasia (language/communication problems), visual impairment, and one-sided paralysis. (Figure 2 shows major centers in the brain that may be damaged by stroke).

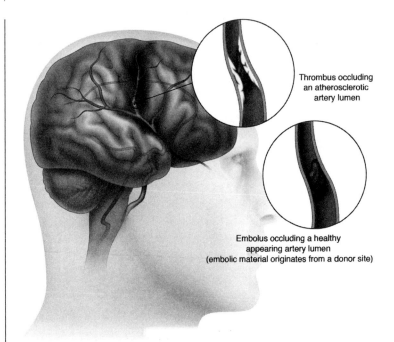

Thrombus occluding
an atherosclerotic
artery lumen

Embolus occluding a healthy
appearing artery lumen
(embolic material originates from a donor site)

Figure 1. Dry (Ischemic) stroke showing thrombus occluding a branch of the middle cerebral artery

Illustration by Thom Graves, © Thom Graves.

"Excess blood" in a given area of the brain is the consequence of wet strokes. This type of stroke is caused by rupture of the blood vessel wall (Fig. 3). These wet strokes are usually more severe than dry strokes.

Remarkably, up to 80% of all strokes are preventable, and for this reason it is important for everyone to ask the question: "Am I at risk?" (Table 1) Most strokes are caused by treatable medical conditions (such as Anna's high blood pressure—see Tables 2a & 2b) that are not being effectively treated. For example, high blood pressure—the leading risk factor for stroke—has been defined in the medical literature by the "rule

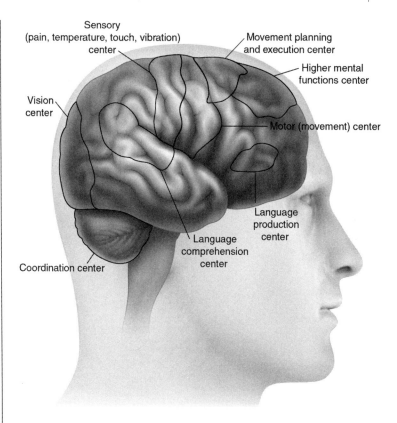

Figure 2. Major Centers of the Brain

Illustration by Thom Graves, © Thom Graves.

of halves": in half of those who have high blood pressure, it is undetected; in half of those who have been diagnosed, it is untreated; and in half of those with high blood pressure that is treated, it is uncontrolled. Table 3 shows a list of common risk factors for stroke, and Figure 4 shows the "big 5" risk factors for stroke. Anna had three of the "big 5"—high blood pressure, diabetes, and tobacco smoking. It is important to note that second-hand smoke may also raise the risk of stroke. The effect of second-hand smoke was glaring in a study conducted in Scotland before and

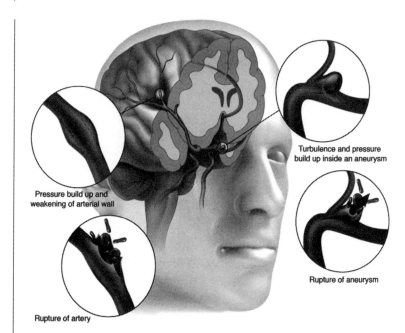

Turbulence and pressure
build up inside an aneurysm

Pressure build up and
weakening of arterial wall

Rupture of aneurysm

Rupture of artery

Figure 3. Wet (hemorrhagic) Stroke

Illustration by Thom Graves, © Thom Graves.

Table 1. Determining Your Risk for Stroke

Factor	Score Card (1 Point for Each Category that Applies)
Age > 45 (men)	1
Age > 55 (women)	
Family history of stroke at any age in mother, father, grandparent, or sibling, or family history of heart attack in father or brother under age 55 or in mother or sister under age 65	1

(continued)

Table 1. (*continued*)

Prior stroke or TIA (transient ischemic attack or ministroke), peripheral artery disease, carotid artery disease, sickle cell disease	1
Blood pressure above 140/90 mmHg, a diagnosis of high blood pressure, taking medications to control blood pressure	1
Tobacco smoker or frequent exposure to tobacco smoke (e.g., by spouse)	1
Overweight: waist circumference of > 35 inches in women and > 40 inches in men or body mass index of > 30[a]	1
Diabetes	1
High cholesterol level (total cholesterol > 200, LDL cholesterol > 100, HDL cholesterol < 40)	1
Irregular heartbeat or atrial fibrillation, heart condition of any kind	1
TOTAL POSSIBLE SCORE	9
A score of 2 or greater *indicates that you may be at elevated risk for stroke and need to visit a doctor for further evaluation and risk reduction interventions.*	

[a] *An easy-to-use BMI calculator can be found at the National Institute of health website: http://www.nhlbisupport.com/bmi/*

Table 2a. Determining Your Blood Pressure

Blood Pressure Category	Systolic Pressure (mmHg) (the Top Number Shown on a Digital Blood Pressure Machine)	Diastolic Pressure (mmHg) (the Bottom Number Shown on a Digital Blood Pressure Machine)
Normal	120 and below	80 and below
Prehypertension	120–139	80–89
Stage 1 hypertension	140–159	90–99
Stage 2 hypertension	160 and above	100 and above

Table 2b. Important Facts about High Blood Pressure

Facts

High blood pressure is known as "the silent killer" because it usually has no signs or symptoms at the time of discovery.

A medical professional can diagnose high blood pressure easily and quickly.

Anyone, even children, can have high blood pressure.

High blood pressure can be prevented by maintaining a healthy lifestyle, including good nutrition and regular exercise.

Effective treatment of high blood pressure with medications can prevent stroke and save your life.

Table 3. Common Treatable Risk Factors for Stroke

Risk Factors	Explanation
High blood pressure	See Table 2
Diabetes mellitus	A fasting blood glucose level of 126mg/dl or greater measured on two occasions. [Note that high blood pressure is more common in individuals with diabetes than those who do not have diabetes].
Obesity	A body mass index (normal 18.5–24.9) greater than 30 (BMI calculator can be found at http://www.nhlbisupport.com/bmi/) or waist circumference greater than 40 inches (102 cm) in men, and greater than 35 inches (88 cm) in women.
High cholesterol	A total cholesterol level of greater than 200 mg/dl, or an LDL "bad" cholesterol level greater than 100 mg/dl. A *low* HDL "good" cholesterol less than 40mg/dl is also a risk factor. "LDL" is the main source of cholesterol build-up in arteries, and "HDL" is responsible for preventing cholesterol build-up in arteries.
Metabolic syndrome	This syndrome is a cluster of conditions linked by insulin resistance. They include high blood pressure, high blood glucose, obesity, high blood triglyceride levels, and/or low HDL cholesterol levels.
Heart disease and atrial fibrillation	Irregular heartbeat (atrial fibrillation), disease of the heart blood vessels (coronary artery disease), heart failure, diseases of the heart valves, having a large "hole" or PFO (patent foramen ovale) in the heart.

(*continued*)

Table 3. (*continued*)

Risk Factors	Explanation
High blood levels of homocysteine	This is an amino acid that is synthesized by the body. Elevated levels may be caused by deficiencies of vitamins B6, B12, and folic acid or acquired genetically.
Disorders of blood clotting	These are usually inherited but may be acquired through certain medical conditions such as lupus, cancer, and HIV. [Rarely, the triad of high estrogen-containing oral contraception, smoking, and migraine with aura may also raise the risk of stroke.]
Sleep apnea	A disorder of sleep characterized by loud snoring and pauses in breathing of more than 10 seconds.
Tobacco smoking	This may include exposure to second-hand tobacco smoke.
Physical inactivity	"Couch potato" or less than 30 minutes per day of moderate intensity activity such as brisk walking, climbing stairs, swimming, and jogging.
Poor diet and nutrition	Too much salt: more than 1 teaspoon (2300 mg) a day or more than ½ teaspoon per day if you have high blood pressure. Note: more than 1000 mg or ½ teaspoon of salt in certain individuals can raise blood pressure numbers by 5 points. High intake of fatty foods.
Excessive alcohol consumption	No more than 1 drink per day for women and 2 drinks per day for men are recommended. One drink is defined as 12 oz of beer, 5oz of wine, 1½ oz of spirits.

(*continued*)

Table 3. (*continued*)

Cocaine abuse (and amphetamine-containing drugs)	All forms of cocaine ingestion including snorting, injecting, and smoking. Amphetamine-containing drugs of abuse such as "Ecstasy" also raise the risk of stroke.
Estrogen replacement therapy (ERT)	This treatment is used to increase estrogen levels in postmenopausal women or in those with early menopause. Because ERT increases the risk of stroke slightly, the risks and benefits should be discussed with your doctor.
Psychological distress	This has been implicated by epidemiological studies in stroke, although it remains controversial. [It is important to note that stress-relieving interventions have been shown to reduce heart attacks, but this is yet to be demonstrated in stroke.]

after the implementation of smoke-free legislation. People who had never smoked reported a significant decrease in exposure to second-hand smoke, which was confirmed by meaningful declines in blood concentrations of contine—a marker of exposure. Moreover, 67% of an overall decrease in the number of admissions for heart attacks associated with this smoke-free legislation occurred in nonsmokers.

Prevention and modification of stroke risk factors begin with changes in certain lifestyle habits, but these require knowledge and a sustainable dose of motivation.

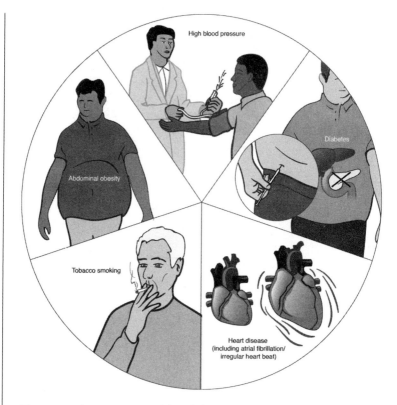

Figure 4. The "Big 5" treatable risk factors for stroke

Illustration by Thom Graves, © Thom Graves.

Here are a few stroke prevention tips that deal with lifestyle changes:

- *Always read food labels during grocery shopping.*

- *Reduce salt intake to less than 1 teaspoon per day (approx 2,300 mg sodium). Instead of table salt, use fresh herbs to add flavor to food. Avoid high-salt meats such as frankfurters, bacon, ham, sausage, luncheon meats, and smoked meats. Canned foods should also be avoided because they are often high in salt content. For individuals with certain medical conditions such as high blood pressure or heart failure, reduce to half a teaspoon of salt per day. Check nutrition labels for the word sodium—a code word for salt (sodium alginate, sodium benzoate, sodium bicarbonate, monosodium glutamate). Excess salt may adversely raise an individual's blood pressure.*

- *Increasing fruit and vegetable consumption to at least five servings per day may reduce the risk of stroke. (For fruits, one serving is: 1 piece of fruit or wedge slice of melon or ¾ cup of 100% fruit juice or ½ cup of canned fruit. For vegetables, one serving is: 1 cup of tossed salad or ½ cup of cooked vegetable.) Fresh fruits and vegetables are potassium rich. (A low blood potassium level—common in individuals taking diuretic blood pressure medications—has been linked to increased stroke risk.)*

- *Increase consumption of fish, poultry, and whole grains. Fish is also a good source of omega-3-fatty acids, which may reduce the risk of stroke. Salmon is the richest source of omega-3-fatty acids, followed by herring, sardines, halibut, and tuna.*

- *Consider increasing intake of soy, fresh tomato, walnuts, almonds, green tea, Korean ginseng tea, and jasmine tea.*

- *Consider a traditional Mediterranean diet. Adherence to this diet significantly reduces the risk of stroke. A Mediterranean diet consists of: olive oil as the main source of monounsaturated fat, reduced red meat, moderate amounts of fish, lots of fruits and vegetables, reduced eggs and dairy products, bread, cereals, potatoes, beans, nuts, seeds, low-to-moderate amount of wine.*

- *Reduce saturated fats, trans fats and total fats (examples are: beef, beef fat, lard, poultry fat, cream, egg yolk (no more than three per week), whole and 2% milk, cheese, coconut oil, palm oil).*

- *Minimize frying foods: broil, bake, grill, roast, or boil instead.*

- *Reduce sweets and sugar-containing beverages (note: ½ gallon of regular soda contains 72 teaspoons of sugar).*

- *Attempt at least 30 minutes of moderate-intensity physical activity five or more times per week (brisk walking suffices, and some individuals, especially stroke survivors with residual disability, may need special exercise equipment or medically supervised programs). For people who cannot find 30 minutes in a day, even three chunks of 10-minute exercising is sufficient. A pedometer attached to the waist with a daily minimum goal of 10,000 steps per day may also help achieve daily physical activity goals. Exercise significantly reduces the risk of stroke and has been shown to improve blood vessel function, although this latter benefit is lost once exercise is stopped. Exercise also raises the "good" cholesterol (HDL-cholesterol), which confers cardiovascular protection at high blood levels.*

- *If you don't drink, don't start. Otherwise, limit alcohol consumption to no more than two drinks per day for most men and one drink/day for women and lighter-weight persons (one drink = 12 oz beer, 5 oz wine, or 1.5 oz spirits).*

- *If you smoke, stop. Consider a medically supervised smoking cessation program. Learn strategies to cope with cravings and relapses. Due to the antianxiety properties of nicotine, it is important to seek a smoking cessation program that not only addresses the physical addiction but also behavioral addiction.*

- *Identify your stress triggers and find a way to manage them. If you have difficulty coping, seek professional help. Do not allow feelings of anxiety or depression to fester.*

- *Attend all scheduled physician visits including an annual physical.*

- *Keep medications visible and post reminders. Use a pillbox and keep medication logs. Plan ahead for refills and try to use only one pharmacy.*

The Man Who Did Not Take His Medicine

Pedro was lying on the bathroom floor next to the toilet bowl. Water was still running from rusty faucets, overflowing the sink, and pooling around his body, as he lay limp on wet porcelain tiles. Lucy was standing over him and whining. The young black Labrador retriever had not left her owner's side since the previous night. It was as if she had predicted it, as if she was responding to some perceptible physiological precursor to Pedro's stroke—a subtle change in his body, perhaps even a "stroke odor" that her heightened sense of smell allowed her to detect. Lucy had followed him everywhere; she lay awake next to him throughout the night, constantly licking the left side of his body. She rushed after him into the bathroom that morning, before Pedro's world began to tilt—the visual metamorphosis, tilting up to180° in seconds, and developing into a violent vertigo that caused him to slump to the ground, hitting his head against the toilet bowl on the way down.

It was 5:30 a.m. The sun had just begun its ascent above the coastline when Pedro woke up to brush his teeth. And now, hours later, he could not get up off the floor. He could not move his left arm or left leg, and he could not feel Lucy licking his left palm. When he realized what was happening, fear filled his soul like a poisonous gas causing a great panic inside him. Dazed and desperate, Pedro dragged himself into the bedroom, sliding onto the wooden floor with his wet clothes, snaking himself around a large floor cushion, knocking over the standing lamp, dragging himself towards the far window by his bed, towards the sunrays that filtered through half-open blinds. Lucy began barking; Pedro began banging against the window. He cried out for help, thumping the glass with his one working arm, trying to alarm his neighbors or anyone who could have saved him. As Lucy barked louder, the stroke tightened its grip, claiming Pedro against his will, pulling the prize right out of him—a piece of his brain—against the tugging of a frantic soul.

Perhaps death is not deaf after all. Perhaps there are times when death can be frightened away. As Pedro cried out for help, banging against his bedroom window, as Lucy barked louder than she had ever done before, something strange began to happen. It was as though the stroke was departing, releasing its grip from Pedro's brain, and slipping into the wind that blew through small cracks that had appeared in the window.

Pedro began moving his left arm and his left leg. He could feel Lucy licking him. He could feel the cut above his left brow, which he sustained from the fall, and the blood trickling down his cheek. He could feel his wet clothes from the overflowing sink, and he was filled with indescribable relief.

I met Pedro shortly after he arrived at the stroke center. Even though he was completely back to normal, his neighbor had convinced him to go to the hospital.

"You had a TIA," I said, "a transient ischemic attack or ministroke."

Pedro was in his mid-forties and he maintained an athletic figure. He seemed distracted, agitated, not fully engaging me, even as I explained what had happened to him, even as I told him the results of the tests that he had undergone. Pedro's brain scans and preliminary blood tests were normal. The only abnormality detected was an irregular heartbeat (atrial fibrillation), which was confirmed by an electrocardiogram.

"I know about that doc. I was diagnosed with irregular heartbeat last year and was given a pill that I gave up on. I think it was called warfarin. There were too many do's and don'ts, and too many blood tests I had to keep taking. They told me that I could bleed if I hit my head or if I fell down because the pill made my blood real thin. I work in construction, doc, and us folks get knocks all the time." After a brief pause, Pedro continued, "I need to get home to my dog. She's all alone and hasn't eaten today."

Eventually, Pedro signed himself out of the hospital against medical advice.

There was nothing I could do or say to stop him, and he declined the help of social services.

When Pedro arrived at his apartment entrance, Lucy's exuberant barking could be heard through the door. It was a great reunion, full of love and affection. Lucy did not leave Pedro's side for the remainder of that day. After cleaning up the debris of the morning chaos, Pedro gave Lucy her favorite food to eat. Together, they played on the floor and on the bed, and later that evening, Lucy chased him around a traffic cone in Morningside Park. Pedro felt alive—bursting with joy as he ran around in circles with his four-legged friend.

Later that night, Lucy began acting strange again. She became restless and clingy, the way she had been the night before. She refused to drink water and became unusually aggressive when Pedro entered the bathroom without her. Sensing her anxiety, Pedro concluded that Lucy's behavior was related to the trauma of the earlier events. He began to gently caress her coat and then cuddled up against her before falling into a deep sleep on the large floor cushion, forgetting to take the pills he was given that morning.

Then, the unfathomable occurred, appearing like a bad dream. When Pedro awoke, Lucy was lying on top of his right leg, fast asleep. When he tried to remove his leg from under Lucy's belly, he realized that he could not do it. He could not even wriggle his toes. The indescribable relief of yesterday was surpassed by sheer fear. Terrified, he excavated his senses in search of buried hope, but the only thing he uncovered was more and more fear. While Pedro and Lucy were asleep, the stroke had returned to steal a piece of his left brain—the opposite side from its last attack—causing Pedro's speech to fail and his right limbs to turn flaccid.

And now Pedro was lying on the same stretcher he had occupied when he had signed himself out of the hospital the previous day. It was his second stroke in less than 48 hours, and a more severe form. Lucy had saved his life. Her loud barking had woken up the neighbor who called 911.

SIX MONTHS LATER...

Pedro spent 2 months on my stroke unit and was then discharged to a rehabilitation hospital. During his rehabilitation, Pedro barely spoke to anyone. Even though he had regained his speech and partial use of his right arm and leg, he barely said much or did much. And now that he was home, his apathy grew. His only social activity was his daily trip to the animal shelter. Accompanied by his home attendant, Pedro visited Lucy at the shelter everyday—a trip he made with his new electric wheelchair. Lucy had lost weight, perhaps even more than her owner. She had lost her appetite and no longer desired play. Instead, she slept throughout most of the day, only to awaken when Pedro visited her, when she would lie awake at the back of her kennel and look at him with long sad eyes that implored him to take her home.

According to a Japanese proverb, a journey of a thousand miles begins with a single step. That morning in my office, after countless visits with me, Pedro decided to open up for the very first time.

"I can't take care of Lucy anymore doc."

It was a powerful step—a courageous beginning on a journey of a thousand miles, and all I needed to do was listen. Sometimes that is all we need to do.

Pedro looked down and began scratching his right arm.

"I get these tingling sensations down my arm and I don't feel myself scratching. Look at these scars, doc."

Pedro lifted up his right arm with his left hand to show me the excoriation marks on his skin.

"I look at myself and I'm not the same person I used to be. People stare at me on the bus and they make me feel uncomfortable. They feel sorry for me, doc. I see the pity in their eyes. I should have taken my medicine, then I wouldn't be like this."

Using my body language, I encouraged Pedro to continue.

"I see it in Lucy's eyes, too, doc, and I can't bear it. I can't stand being apart from her. I should have taken my medicine, doc."

There is a time for every emotion and every deed—even misery. And there are moments in life when we are lost in such times. As I traveled with Pedro through his underworld of depression, we seemed to be going around in circles. Was there a dream I could give him that revealed a way out? Was there a way to bend time around his pain and reveal better days? But this was a time to be silent, to lend him my ear, to listen to Pedro's footsteps on his private journey to recovery, and to learn from the greatest physician of us all—Time.

ONE YEAR LATER...

Lucy was wagging her tail—an effusive expression of her delight as she chased after the ball that Pedro had just thrown with his restored right arm. They were in Morningside Park at the bottom of a hillside near a newly planted tree. Thousands of daffodils were in bloom—their golden-yellow petals glistened in the sunlight, covering the field like an impressionist painting. Pedro had found a way out. He had found a way to bend time around his pain and see his better days. He had fallen many times, but kept getting up, moving forward, step-by-step, mile-by-mile, on the road to his recovery. And now he felt whole again, running around in circles, hurling the ball with his restored right arm, bursting with joy as he played on the grass with his four-legged friend.

Comment

The warning signs and symptoms of stroke are not exclusive to stroke, but the manner in which they appear typically is. Stroke symptoms are not insidious and do not classically progress over days, weeks, or months. When they strike, they do so suddenly, and without warning. Cardinal symptoms of stroke include: sudden numbness or weakness in one or both sides of the body; sudden difficulty speaking, understanding speech, or confusion; sudden loss of vision in one or both eyes; sudden dizziness, incoordination, or loss of balance; and sudden severe headache with no known cause (Fig. 5).

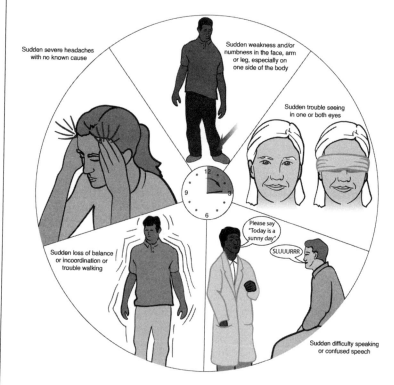

Figure 5. Cardinal stroke warning symptoms or signs (remember: call 911!)
Illustration by Thom Graves, © Thom Graves.

Transient ischemic attacks (TIA) or transient stroke symptoms that resolve completely within 24 hours may be warning signs of worse things to come—we saw this outcome after Pedro's initial transient stroke symptoms. Indeed, about 15% of people who have a stroke report a history of TIA. Approximately 5% of people who experience a TIA will have a full-blown stroke within 48 hours, and approximately 11% will experience one within 90 days. And when other adverse events following a TIA are included, such as death or cardiovascular events, the number of people with subsequent afflictions following a TIA rises to 25% within 90 days. In many countries, people experiencing TIAs are not admitted into the hospital. Instead, these individuals are referred to a "weekly" TIA clinic. But securing a clinic appointment has been shown to take an average of 9 days from referral to appointment. In one analysis performed on 210 consecutive patients referred with suspected TIA to a weekly clinic, 11 patients (5.2%) had a full-blown stroke before their appointment came, 9 of which caused significant disability. For these reasons, people with transient stroke symptoms should be evaluated with the same urgency as those with persistent stroke symptoms. Table 4 shows the risk of stroke following a TIA at specific time points.

*The risk of **recurrent** stroke after an initial full-blown stroke is up to 24% in women and up to 42% in men, within 5 years. However, this rate of recurrent stroke varies depending on the cause of the stroke. For example, the **1-year** rate of recurrent stroke in patients whose stroke is caused by atrial fibrillation is approximately 15%. Fortunately, these risks can be minimized with targeted treatment of predisposing medical and*

Table 4. Estimated Risk of a Full-Blown Stroke After a TIA (Transient Ischemic Attack or Ministroke or Take Immediate Action)

Time Point Following TIA	Risk of Full-Blown Stroke (%)
30 days	4–8
1 year	12–13
5 years	24–29

behavioral conditions (Table 5), and antistroke drugs that have been proven to reduce the risk of recurrent stroke (Table 6). Pedro's TIA and recurrent stroke were caused by atrial fibrillation (irregular heartbeat) and failure to take his medicines. Atrial fibrillation is a treatable and common cause of stroke that can be diagnosed by checking your own pulse to detect any irregular rhythm or with a simple painless test called an electrocardiogram, which only takes a few minutes to perform (Table 7 shows the basic tests that need to be performed on stroke patients). The symptoms of atrial fibrillation are not specific because they overlap with several other conditions. They include:

- Fluttering sensations in the chest, palpitations, or jumping of the heart

- Dizziness, light-headedness, feeling faint

- Weak pulse, irregular pulse, racing pulse, or pulse that feels too slow

- Shortness of breath with exertion, fatigue

- Chest pain, chest tightness

- [For additional information: www.StopAfib.org is a patient-to-patient resource specifically for patients with atrial fibrillation and their families.]

Because atrial fibrillation is intermittent (paroxysmal atrial fibrillation) in 25% of individuals who have it, extended electrocardiographic monitoring (24–48 hours) is often required to detect it, and in some cases up to 21 days of mobile outpatient cardiac monitoring is performed. Ineffective irregular quivering of the upper chamber or "atria" of the heart characterizes it, rather than the normal regular and robust beating required to pump blood through the heart. This results in pooling and stagnation of blood inside the heart and the formation of blood clots (thrombus). These blood clots may break up, releasing pieces into the bloodstream that may travel to the brain and cause a "dry" stroke by blocking random arteries.

Table 5. Disease-Specific Methods to Reduce the Risk of Another Stroke

Risk Factor	Treatment
High blood pressure	A comprehensive approach involves health nutrition, daily exercise, maintaining a healthy weight (body mass index 18.5–24.9), and antihypertensive medications to attain blood pressure targets below 120/80.
Diabetes	Lower fasting glucose blood levels to 126 mg/dl. Maintain blood levels of Hemoglobin A1c to ≤7%. Everyone with diabetes MUST know their A1c number and what A1c means. [For more information on A1c, visit http://diabetesa1c.org/] If changes in diet, increased exercise, and weight loss do not work, drug therapy is indicated. High blood pressure is more common among diabetic individuals than nondiabetic individuals, so this must also be rigorously controlled (blood pressure should be maintained below 130/80 mmHg).
High cholesterol	There are three pillars for lowering cholesterol: (1) Diet: Eat foods low in saturated fat such as fat-free or 1% milk, fish, skinless chicken, lean meats, fruits and vegetables, and whole-grain foods. Limit egg yolks, full-fat dairy products, liver, and organ meats. Increase soluble fiber (lowers LDL cholesterol) such as fruits (oranges, apples, pears), vegetables (carrots, Brussels sprouts), oats, barley, flax seed, nuts. (2) Exercise: at least 30 minutes of sweat-breaking physical activity on all or most days (lowers LDL cholesterol and raises HDL cholesterol)

(*continued*)

Table 5. (*continued*)

Risk Factor	Treatment
	(3) Cholesterol-lowering medications: Discuss optimal choice with your physician.
Atrial fibrillation	Rate control drugs, rhythm control drugs, and blood thinners (warfarin) Surgical ablation or catheter ablation may also be performed for certain patients.
Carotid stenosis (serious narrowing of a segment of the carotid artery in the neck through which blood reaches the brain)	Individuals with high-grade stenosis (more than 70% and less than 100% of the blood vessel lumen is occluded) and have had a stroke or TIA should have carotid endarterectomy (surgical reopening) if there are no medical contraindications. In the case of individuals in whom surgery is deemed too risky, carotid artery stents may be inserted instead. The decision to perform surgery on an individual who has not had a stroke or TIA (usually discovered incidentally during screening) should be made on a case-by-case basis and carefully weighed against the risks of the procedure, since the benefit of carotid surgery in this group of people is small.
Blood clot (thrombus) inside the heart	Treatment with warfarin
Sickle cell disease	Stroke caused by sickle cell disease should be treated with "exchange" blood transfusions.

(*continued*)

Table 5. (*continued*)

Obesity	Weight reduction has benefits that extend well beyond lowering stroke risk. It lowers blood pressure and blood sugar, lowers cholesterol, reduces body aches and pains, improves sleep, improves breathing, and increases energy levels. Determine your body mass index, waist circumference, and weight and compare these numbers with normal values (Table 3). Determine your daily caloric requirement (personal calorie requirement calculators are commercially available, free calorie calculators are available on the Internet, or ask your doctor), and try not to exceed this number. An extra 300 calories per day—such as from salty snacks, soft drinks, and increased meal sizes—will add one pound of fat to your body every 12 days. *Remember extra calories, regardless of their source, are stored in the body as fat*. Weight loss should be gradual and realistic goals should be set. Supervised weight loss programs may also help. Note: According to the 2008 CIA World Factbook, the Japanese are one of three nations with the longest life expectancy in the world (The United States is ranked #45). The Japanese have a proverb that says: If you stop eating when your stomach is 80% full, you will have little need to visit the doctor.
Tobacco smoking	Stop smoking and avoid second hand smoke. Smoking cessation programs that address physical addiction AND behavioral addiction are recommended. Call 1-800-QUIT-NOW for the phone quitline in your state (for United States residents).

Table 6. Antistroke Drugs for the Prevention of Recurrent Stroke

Drug	Dosage
Aspirin[a]	50–325 mg once a day
Clopidogrel	75 mg/day once a day
Aspirin plus extended-release dipyridamole	25 mg/200 mg twice a day
Warfarin	Dosage is adjusted until a therapeutic serum level is attained, as measured by blood coagulation tests called prothrombin time and international normalized ratio (INR). For stroke prevention, the INR range is usually maintained between 2 and 3.
Cholesterol-lowering "statin" drugs such as atorvastatin	80 mg once a day (recommended dose for atorvastatin in people who have already had a "dry" stroke)

[a]*Some patients may have strokes despite being on aspirin therapy because of "Aspirin Resistance," although more common reasons are poor medication compliance, and interaction with ibuprofen or naproxen. Genetic variations may be responsible for aspirin resistance.*

Table 7. Basic Tests that Should Be Performed on Everyone with a Stroke or TIA (Transient Ischemic Attack)

Test	Description
Blood tests	Fasting blood glucose, serum electrolytes, creatinine, complete blood count, full cholesterol blood panel, blood coagulation studies
Brain scans	Computer tomography (CT) scan or magnetic resonance imaging (MRI)
Carotid artery imaging	Doppler ultrasound or magnetic resonance angiography of the neck vessels or CT angiography of the neck vessels.
Heart tests	Electrocardiogram, echocardiogram

A Wise Man Fails to Recognize the Signs

Rude and crude, an uninvited intruder, Mr. Stroke.
A battering ram assaulting me into submission,
humiliation.
I am reduced to a heaving flood of tears—
born of my pain.
It is unrelenting,
inducing a metaphysical vertigo,
conversations with self,
bewildering, confounding—
Kafkaesque moments, existential meanderings.
Why me again?
And then suddenly there is fight in me,
suddenly a new drive to live rages in me.
Right here, under this oppressive blanket of loneliness and misery,
I will fight this beast.
I will be unrelenting,
and I will walk again
I will dance again
I will sing again.
To new tomorrows—healthier tomorrows.

Written by Omar.

Two years later his second stroke brought him to his knees. It was a fierce attack, reminiscent of his previous TIA. His symptoms began with pins-and-needle sensations of his left cheek and left hand, followed by weakness of his entire left side. Omar thought that his symptoms would go away the way they did the last time if he lay down to rest. So he did not call 911. He did not appreciate the urgency of his symptoms—the window of opportunity, and the need to act fast. By the time he woke up from his nap, millions of brain cells had been killed. His stroke signs had worsened to the point where he could not swallow his own saliva, which constantly drooled from the left corner of his mouth. He could not generate enough force to make an audible grunt, and he was too weak to rise up from the sofa upon which he slumped. The telephone was less than 4 feet away, but Omar could not reach it no matter how hard he tried. Then, with a great heave, he slid onto the carpet but lacked the strength to roll over towards the telephone. All he could do was lie there. He spent 3 days and 3 nights lying on the floor of his apartment soaked in urine and feces. Each time the phone rang, hope would appear, only to disappear as hours went by and no one came to save him as he slipped into a deepening coma.

No one on earth has been promised tomorrow, just as no one could have predicted whether Omar would survive. The dice of life and death tumbles in the heavens, and no one on earth knows how it will land.

Half of Omar's brain did not make it alive, but the other half survived, thanks to his concerned daughter who finally showed up when she could not reach Omar by telephone.

It was not my medicine, but something else that sustained Omar during those early hospital days. I watched as nurses poured liquid food through a thin tube in his nose, which ran all the way down the back of his throat to his stomach. I watched them suction out the copious secretions that clogged his breathing tube through a hoselike device, which was connected to a machine on the wall. I watched as they turned him each day, and cleaned his wrinkled skin with a tepid sponge. I helped to change his full bag of urine into which a rubber catheter emptied contents directly from his bladder. I saw his daughter's grief—her daily mourning at his bedside. And even though he was too sick to watch, I helped to change the channel of his television set to his favorite station before I left his room.

After a few weeks of this, Omar became stronger. The tubes, which pierced his body, had been removed, and his daughter smiled at me for the very first time.

"It is not my time," Omar told his daughter as he emerged from his coma.

For 3 days and 3 nights, this 80-year-old man had wrestled with death on his living room floor. He had pushed back even harder on his hospital bed, and he had won.

Omar's strokes were caused by high-grade carotid artery stenosis—a critical narrowing of the carotid artery in his right neck caused by accumulation of fatty deposits of cholesterol loaded cells within inflamed arterial walls called plaques (Fig. 6). And because this artery feeds Omar's right brain, his two strokes shared similar left-sided symptoms (although the first attack was transient in nature). Omar was considered to be too high a risk for surgical opening of the narrowed carotid artery—a procedure called *carotid endarterectomy,* which involves placing a temporary clamp on both sides of the narrowed diseased segment of the artery while the artery is opened, so that the inner core of fatty plaques and clot material is cleaned out. His old age in combination with other medical conditions such as heart disease and high blood cholesterol made him a risky candidate for major surgery. Instead, he underwent an alternative second-choice procedure called *carotid stenting,* which involves insertion of an expandable mechanical sleeve or "stent" into the diseased segment of the artery through a catheter, and then expanding it until the arterial lumen is wide open; it is then left there to keep the artery open and to maintain the restored normal blood flow to his right brain. But the real cost of his stroke could not be restored—an unusual pattern of paralysis that spared only his right arm, which he would raise with great pride whenever I entered his room.

"I wrote another poem today," he would say, pen in hand.

One day, during my daily rounds, I asked Omar for the secret of his strength—how he managed to stay so strong despite his severe stroke, how he managed to be so positive, where most would be demoralized.

"I found a rose," he said, "I found a rose in the center of my soul."

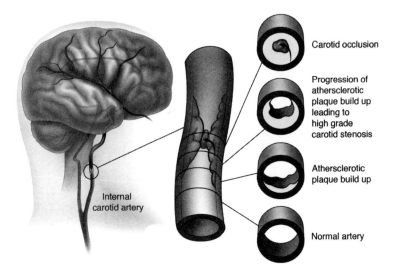

Figure 6. Carotid artery disease

Illustration by Thom Graves, © Thom Graves.

The silence that followed was filled with a tranquility that can only be found in paradise. And yet I was in a hospital, holding the hand of a stroke-stricken man.

"Find yours," he continued, "find the center of your soul, and when you do, you will find the answer to your question."

That moment left a strong impression in my heart, which is still with me today. In a short period of time, Omar had shared timeless stories with me. He talked of signs in our universe, which "many view as coincidences"—the solstices and equinoxes, the different cycles of the Earth around the sun, and the meaning of vivid dreams. I discovered the "Solar Hejri," an ancient Persian calendar that is still used today. I learned about Eastern philosophy through the words of Osho[1]: "The whole Eastern methodology can be reduced to one word—witnessing. The whole Western methodology can be reduced to one word—analyzing. With analyzing, you go round and around. Witnessing simply gets you out of the circle."

---

[1] Osho, Awareness: *The Key to Living in Balance.* New York: St. Martin's Griffin, 2001.

"Do not overanalyze, doc," he would say. Omar believed that we must shed our old skin, "the way a snake does"—we must separate ourselves from old problems so that they do no harm our present moment in time. But perhaps his finest words were his reflections on love, his comment that the quality of life is not measured by health or wealth or the scope of man's works, but by the amount of love that bathes his soul.

"This is the only meaningful thing in life," he said, "but love is much more than a feeling; it is an action." Omar told me that it is the act of loving that can drive out all the fear and suffering in the world.

After 3 months with Omar, it was time for us to say goodbye. As I watched Omar depart like an old sage on a rolling hospital stretcher, I remembered our conversations about the *"Power of Myth"* (Omar was a big fan of the author Joseph Campbell), and I replayed our exchanges on signs and coincidences. I could not understand how a man so wise failed to recognize the warning signs of his own body during his initial stroke symptoms. Why did he choose a nap over calling 911? I remembered him telling me that wisdom is "transformed knowledge," and I thought of all my other highly educated patients who also chose a nap over calling 911.

As Omar approached the exit doors, he asked the patient escorts to stop so that he could look back at me one last time. When he smiled and waved at me with his right hand, I felt as though I was being singled out from among the crowd in a royal procession.

"To new tomorrows, my friend," he said, "to healthier tomorrows."

The arms of stroke are strong: its rigid embrace is hard to unfold. Stiff elbows become chains that often disable a hug or simple handshake. Yet on nights when I visit ex-patients in my sleep, I often come across Omar. He is standing in the center of an empty room, arm-in-arm with his shadow, holding a crimson rose, and dancing to silent music before an entranced audience of cells inside my brain. When I open my eyes, it is a new tomorrow—a new day within which "will" explodes into a chorus of optimism that presages victory: He will walk again, he will dance again, he will sing again.

Comment

In December 1995, there was a paradigm shift in the treatment of stroke. The clot-buster or t-PA (tissue plasminogen activator) became the first weapon in our arsenal against stroke (Fig. 7). But our response must be swift; it must begin within 3 hours from the onset of stroke symptoms in order to forestall the type of regional brain damage that befell Omar, and reduce disability.

Restoration of blood flow to the brain after a stroke is called reperfusion, and thrombolysis is a term used to describe the counterattack or dissolution of the offending blood clots. At the time this book was written, intravenous t-PA, injected through peripheral veins in the limbs, was the

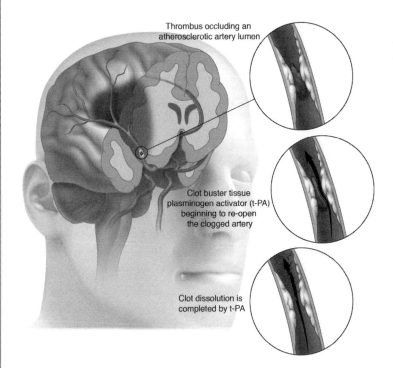

Thrombus occluding an atherosclerotic artery lumen

Clot buster tissue plasminogen activator (t-PA) beginning to re-open the clogged artery

Clot dissolution is completed by t-PA

Figure 7. The mechanism action of clot-buster tissue plasminogen activator (t-PA)

Illustration by Thom Graves, © Thom Graves.

only drug approved by the U.S. Food and Drug Administration (FDA) for the treatment of ischemic (dry) stroke. It must be administered within a strict 3-hour time window in order to be effective and avoid serious side effects, such as bleeding into the brain. When used properly, t-PA significantly reduces disability from stroke. Indeed, 31% to 50% of patients treated with intravenous t-PA will be left with minimal or zero disability 3 months after receiving this drug.

Until recently, efforts to extend the 3-hour time window for the treatment of ischemic stroke with intravenous t-PA have failed. But in 2008, a European study demonstrated in a select group of patients, which did not include patients over the age of 80 years, those with extremely severe strokes, and those with a combination of previous stroke and diabetes mellitus, that t-PA may be effectively and safely administered between 3 hours and 4.5 hours of stroke symptom onset, although it remains clear that the earlier patients are treated, the better their clinical outcome.

The National Institute of Neurological Disorders and Stroke (NINDS) recommends a target of increasing the number of stroke patients arriving at the hospital within 3 hours to 70% by 2013. Most hospitals in America today have 3-hour arrival rates of stroke patients (from the very first stroke symptom to the time of arrival in the emergency department) well below 50%. Indeed, some patients like Omar try to "sleep off" their neurological symptoms. A major reason for this poor statistic is that public knowledge of stroke symptoms and the need to call 911 immediately is grossly inadequate. However, fixing this knowledge gap, even though this is a logical first step, is not the simple answer—we saw that with Omar during his second stroke, when he chose to take a nap instead of calling 911.

Knowledge, by itself, is not sufficient to bring about behavior change: it needs to be "transformed." This involves personalizing a need for change and inspiring the journey towards it. It involves transforming knowledge into action. There are those who desire change but lack the knowledge of how to get there, and there are those with the knowledge of how to get there but lack the desire for change.

But more than a decade after its approval by the FDA, less than 3% of ischemic stroke patients presenting to American hospitals are treated with t-PA —no wonder stroke remains the leading cause of adult disability in America.

Many reasons have been identified as a cause of the crisis in the number of patients being treated emergently, and most fall into two categories: prehospital and intrahospital delays to emergency stroke treatment. And while the growing stroke center certification program[2] across America has begun to effectively address intrahospital delays by implementing and monitoring rapid assessment protocols for the stroke patient, and mandating 24-hour multidisciplinary stroke teams, the greatest barrier to treatment remains prehospital delays, and the greatest culprit is behavioral: poor recognition of stroke symptoms among the public and failure to

---

[2] The Stroke Center Program: The stroke center certification program is another landmark in the evolution of stroke care and stroke systems in the United States. It is the first major effort to pull together the fragments of care into a cohesive model that delivers comprehensive interventions across the entire continuum of care, which includes stroke prevention, stroke treatment, stroke rehabilitation, and stroke education. In order to become a stroke center, hospitals must fulfill state or federal certification requirements. These include: having a round-the-clock team of physicians (emergency department physicians, neurologists, neurosurgeons, and internists) and nurses with specific training in stroke care, integrating the emergency medical services into stroke training programs and triage protocols, maintaining written care protocols with medical evidence-based guidelines, demonstrating rapid response times for intrahospital triage and evaluation of stroke patients from the point of arrival, including brain-imaging assessment times and blood test turnaround times. Finally, stroke centers must have an organizational structure, which includes a center director, and robust data-driven multidisciplinary quality improvement activities. The benefits of certified stroke centers are numerous and include: increased use of t-PA, increased adherence to medical evidence-based stroke prevention guidelines, better patient outcomes such as decreased odds of death and institutionalized care by 25%, and decreased length of hospital stay for stroke. When a stroke is suspected and 911 is called, most state ambulance networks now have mandatory diversion protocols to bypass noncertified hospitals in favor of certified stroke centers (another reason to call 911). A list of designated stroke centers is available from State Health departments or from the Joint Commission on Accreditation of Healthcare Organizations (JCAHO).

call 911 at their onset. In fact, only one-third of individuals having a stroke are aware of its symptoms, and most bystanders do not recognize its signs. Moreover, individuals with the highest risk and incidence of stroke, including men, African Americans, and people at least 75 years old, remain the least informed about the warning signs of stroke.

In the 2001 Behavioral Risk Factor Surveillance System (BRFSS) survey, only 17.2% were aware of the five cardinal symptoms of stroke and would call 911 if they thought that someone was having a stroke. This crisis in public stroke awareness is finally receiving attention from nonprofit and government organizations, including the National Institute of Neurological Disorders and Stroke, the American Stroke Association, and the National Stroke Association. Several innovative stroke awareness campaigns have emanated from these organizations such as the National Stroke Association's Hip Hop Stroke K-12th grade education program conceived by Diane Mulligan, and of which the author is the Principal Investigator and codeveloper. This program promotes the Cincinnati Stroke Scale used by ambulance personnel to identify stroke victims in the field, as a stroke recognition tool for school children and their parents (Table 8). This easy-to-learn scale, captured in the acronym FAST, was incorporated into a rap song and cartoon created by popular rapper Doug E. Fresh, Ian "Electric" James, and Bill and Colleen Davis in partnership with the author:

- *"F" represents face: ask the person with a suspected stroke to smile, and if one side of the face droops down, a stroke may be occurring.*

- *"A" represents arm: ask the person with a suspected stroke to raise both arms ahead of him or her, and if one arm drifts downwards or if the person is unable to lift one arm, a stroke may be occurring.*

- *"S" represents speech: ask the person with a suspected stroke to repeat a simple sentence such as "the sky is bright blue", and if he or she is unable to correctly repeat the sentence due to slurring or jumbling up of words or is unable to produce any words at all, a stroke may be occurring.*

- *"T" represents time: time to call 911.*

Table 8. The Cincinnati Stroke Scale for Identifying a Stroke (FAST Acronym)

Letter	Meaning
F	FACIAL DROOP: Have individual smile or show teeth and look for an uneven face. Normal: Both sides of the face move equally or not at all. Abnormal: One side of the individuals face droops.
A	ARM WEAKNESS: Have individual close eyes and extend arms with palms up. Look for a drift. Normal: Arms remain extended equally or drift equally or do not move at all. Abnormal: One arm drifts down when compared with the other.
S	SPEECH: Have individual repeat a phrase such as "You can't teach an old dog new tricks." Normal: The phrase is repeated correctly and clearly. Abnormal: The individuals words are slurred or confused or individual is unable to speak.
T	TIME: Time to call 911—must also note time of symptom onset.

A Stroke Saved His Life

"What is bad luck for one man is good luck for another."
Ashanti proverb.

There are no green hills in the ghetto, just heaps of refuse swarming in their innards with rats and buzzing on the outside with overfed flies. There is no view of the mountaintop from the ghetto, just a view of the next decrepit block. Happiness has been held hostage by pain, and no one can afford to pay the ransom. Beggars roam the streets, treading on broken bottles looking for food or a quick fix. Stress and anxiety pollute the air, causing high rates of depression and irrational aggression. Freedom is not on the march here, stroke is—trampling what's left of good health.

"Midnight" had never seen a full moon or watched the sunrise—he was too busy looking over his shoulders. His whole world spanned 10 city blocks where the biggest ambition was to become a mailman or join the military. But there were other role models in his neighborhood: uneducated pimps and drug pushers wearing alligator skin shoes and silk shirts on dingy street corners, with pockets full of blood money.

"I should be pushing up daisies, doc" he told me, "but my stroke saved my life."

I had never heard this before, and as I looked at him, I could not imagine how on earth a stroke so disabling can save anyone's life.

Midnight's real name was Andrew: he was 41 years old. A stroke he suffered 6 years ago left him paralyzed on his right face, arm, and leg. The contractures in his limbs caused a flexion deformity of his slender body, and his speech was slow and slurred. He looked back at me with an uneven smile, realizing that his words had struck a chord, and then he spoke again.

"My stroke is a blessing from above, doc."

At this point I paused and leaned back, filled with curiosity, preparing myself for the story of a life that was liberated by stroke.

Andrew's father died from drug-related homicide when Andrew was still in his mother's womb. His uncle, who is currently serving a life sentence in jail also for drug-related homicide, raised him and his brothers. By the time Andrew was 15, he was well known on the streets—a seasoned truant whose badge of honor was his drug peddling skill. But by the age of 17, Andrew began to fall slowly apart: he had become a drug addict—a victim of his own crime. He would mix heroin and cocaine and inject the solution directly into his veins several times a day. And because his habit is expensive to maintain, it was not long before Andrew began resorting to armed robbery. Over the next decade, he spent most of his life between prison and emergency departments. He became increasingly bipolar—caught in a cycle of drug-induced mania and profound depression. Andrew's mind was disheveled—his skin was mangled by deep disfiguring track marks, which caused keloidal scars. His days consisted of vomiting and passing out on vacant park benches. His nights were the same—more vomiting and passing out, the darkness bringing with it a strange silence that filled him with a suicidal urge.

"I didn't have the guts to shoot myself," he told me, "so I chose madness instead."

Then one day Andrew had a stroke.

As daylight fled with its heat and night arrived in a cool breeze, Andrew searched hard for a vein on his feet. The dirty syringe was filled with an unusually large dose of cocaine mixed with heroin. Within minutes of the injection, Andrew collapsed onto the ground with his eyes turned upwards as if he were in a trance, and his mouth turned sideways as if one side were paralyzed.

Two weeks later Andrew awoke in the intensive care unit of the hospital. He felt as though he had emerged from a monstrous dream and did not know how he got there. The drama of alarms and ventilator beeps was surreal. Andrew had been in a coma for 2 weeks from a malignant stroke. His brain was rescued from fatal swelling in a ferocious battle between life and death. Hyperosmolar brain-shrinking fluids had kept him alive. But there was a price to pay—Andrew had sacrificed the use of his right arm and leg, which were paralyzed. Little did he know that this was the sacrifice that would lead him to a new life.

"I got a second shot at life, doc," he said, "I couldn't shoot dope no more."

Andrew had lost the ability to inject himself. He could not walk, and he could barely communicate. His dominant right hand was immobile and hyperflexed. For 3 months in the hospital, he had no access to drugs or friends who could have helped him administer them.

"I cried everyday all day, doc, and it felt good," he told me, "I would sit by the window and watch the sunrise—I never saw it before, doc."

When it was time to leave the hospital, after an amazing recovery, Andrew did not want to go. He screamed and pleaded not to be discharged to the shelter. Even though he was physically better, the fear of his past still haunted his mind. But Andrew had to leave.

A few weeks later, Andrew went on a field trip with his "Stroke of Hope[1]" support group. They were taken to an ice cream parlor in the suburbs. The bus ride was enthralling, and it was the first time Andrew had traveled out of the city. When they arrived at an ice cream parlor, he was both excited and nervous. People seemed happy wherever he looked. He

---

[1] *Stroke* of Hope is a not-for-profit organization in the United States that provides support for stroke survivors, at *http://www.strokeofhope.net/about.htm*. For more help locating a stroke support group near you, visit the American Stroke Association at *http://www.strokeassociation.org/presenter.jhtml?identifier=3030354* or the National Stroke Association at *http://www.stroke.org/site/PageServer?pagename=support_groups*.

saw couples holding hands and little children laughing aloud. Everyone was polite and friendly, offering a helping hand as he limped towards the seating area on the side of the room. Then he was served his vanilla ice cream.

At this point, Andrew paused in the middle of narrating his story and looked away from me. I remember the teardrops that leaked from his eyes as his emotions swelled. And then he said these words to me:

"While I was on the streets, doc, I would have thousands of dollars in my pocket, but I never in my life felt as happy as that day in the ice cream parlor."

Comment

An anonymous West Coast user coined the phrase, "If coke is a lady, then crack is a bitch." But there is nothing ladylike about causing a stroke. Cocaine in any of its forms (smoked, snorted, or injected) is a well-established risk factor for stroke. When injected concomitantly with heroin, as in Andrew's case, the effects of cocaine remain deadly. Contributing factors to its stroke risk include cocaine's ability to cause massive surges in blood pressure, severe constriction of brain arteries, and alteration of blood clotting properties. The National Institute on Drug Abuse "Monitoring the Future Survey" in 2007 found that by 12th grade, close to 8% of students had used cocaine in some form, and almost half of these students had used crack. And because the scientific literature is populated by cocaine-associated strokes in younger ages, physicians began searching for cocaine metabolites in the urine of young patients with stroke. However, in a case series reported by the author at the 2006 American Academy of Neurology Annual Meeting, older age groups, up to age 79, were also found to have cocaine-associated strokes.

As the use of cocaine waned in the 1990s, other psychostimulants rose to prominence in the United States. Perhaps the most notorious are amphetamines and methamphetamines. Illicit preparations of these substances include "crystal meth," "speed," "uppers," "pep pills," "black beauties," "ice," and "tina." They can be smoked, injected, snorted, and even drunk in beverages ("biker's coffee") with devastating consequences that include stroke. Both "dry" strokes and "wet" strokes have been reported in amphetamine abusers. Severe headaches are usually the earliest symptoms of amphetamine-related stroke, often beginning within minutes of drug ingestion. Dangerous elevations of blood pressures occur and are the presumed basis of amphetamine-related stroke, although irregular narrowing of brain blood vessels associated with inflammation has also been reported (cerebral vasculitis).

Over-the-counter diet pills and cold nasal decongestants containing substances similar to amphetamines (phenylpropanolamine or PPA, and ephedra) have been shown to cause stroke. The U.S. Food and Drug

Administration finally banned PPA- and ephedra-containing products in the years 2000 and 2003, respectively. Despite this ban, it remains prudent for individuals (especially those diagnosed with high blood pressure) to be aware of the substances contained in over-the-counter diet pills and cold nasal decongestants. Some of these substances include ephedrine, pseudoephedrine, fenfluramine, and other amphetamine-like substances that may raise blood pressure levels and increase the risk of stroke.

Heroin abuse can also lead to stroke, although unlike cocaine and amphetamine-associated strokes, the mechanism is more indirect. Intravenous heroin users are at high risk for infections of the heart and heart valves (endocarditis), which may lead to stroke. Heroin overdose may slow breathing rates down to deadly levels, causing insufficient blood pressures required to nourish brain cells, which in turn may lead to stroke. During times of drug shortages, heroin users have been reported to crush narcotic prescription medications (often available in the underground drug trade) and inject these into neck veins, inadvertently puncturing the carotid artery, and introducing particles that may cause stroke (see Episode 10).

While it is important to recognize the relationship between drug abuse and stroke, it should be emphasized that excessive alcohol consumption and tobacco at any dose account for more strokes than do all illicit drugs combined.

A Stroke that Occurred during Sex

It was not long before layers of sweat began accumulating between their interlocked bodies as they made love. Her face was transformed by a glow, as though the sun were rising inside her. They were approaching a place where space and time cease to exist—where minutes are absorbed into infinity and ecstasy is close. She could feel its primitive force quickening the rhythm in her heart. It was nearing. But then she noticed an aching at the back of her head that was intensifying. Gripping him hard, she started to scream in pleasure and pain; a thunderclap headache had struck her brain at the height of it all.

Elizabeth passed out, but Sam, oblivious, continued to thrust.

ONE HOUR LATER...

Chestnut eyes stared out of her frightened face. She could not have been more than 30 years old. As I adjusted the focus of my ophthalmoscope, I saw islands of blood in the back of her eyes called subhyaloid hemorrhages that were clues to a grave diagnosis. Elizabeth had suffered a catastrophic stroke. An aneurysm inside her brain had erupted from the pressure of sexual euphoria and spewed its contents all over her brain. There was blood everywhere and massive brain tissue destruction. It was only a matter of time before the mounting pressure inside her skull would kill off the remaining brain cells. She needed emergent neurosurgery to evacuate the blood clots and clip the burst aneurysm inside her head. Suddenly, in the middle of my physical examination, Elizabeth began convulsing—flailing wildly and causing dangerous pressure surges inside her brain. I treated her with everything modern medicine had to offer: anticonvulsant drugs, intracranial pressure-lowering drips, and "forced" hyperventilation through a high-tech breathing machine. Nothing worked; she got worse, sliding through my grip from stupor to coma.

Down the hall, Elizabeth's body convulsed in her fight to stay alive. In the waiting room, Sam paced up and down clutching his head, his own soul convulsing, trying to survive the wreckage and keep his mind. Everything happened so fast.

There is a point of no return: when the torch of life is handed over to death in the timeless journey of souls. No matter how strong our medicine or heroic our efforts at resuscitation, there is no turning back once the handover is made.

The neurosurgeon did not need to tell me that it was too late to operate on Elizabeth. I already knew. But how would I face Sam?

I stood at the waiting room entrance looking nervously at him. His terror was palpable. I moved towards him to deliver the tragic news.

It was not the first time that I had experienced this: an aneurysm that burst during sex.

It was not the first time that death had invaded a most sacred act of human expression. Nothing is off-limits to stroke—not even the act of lovemaking. It can come at any moment—everything is fair game. Sam felt responsible, asking himself over again, "Would the aneurysm have burst if I hadn't been making love to her?"

ONE WEEK LATER . . .

The sky is blue. Yesterday has been blown away by the wind. I open the back door of my car and hang my white coat on the small handle above the glass. But before I climb into the drivers' seat, my thoughts slip to Elizabeth and Sam. Images of them flood my mind as I gaze through trees that line the horizon. The tide of their story recedes. The sun rises bringing with it a new day.

Comment

The sudden nature of symptoms is the hallmark of any stroke and one that binds the innumerable manifestations of this disease. Brain hemorrhages caused by ruptured aneurysms, a devastating form of stroke, are no different in this regard. They occur abruptly, at any age, at anytime, including during sexual activity or exercise or rest. Most Americans have heard of aneurysms, but few recognize its symptoms or know its risk factors. Aneurysms are abnormal outpouchings from the wall of arteries in the body due to congenital defects or weak spots in their walls (Fig. 3). They can affect any artery including those in the brain and may increase in size over time, increasing the risk of potentially fatal rupture. Other factors that increase the risk of rupture include: a family history of a ruptured aneurysm, high blood pressure, tobacco smoking, and cocaine use. Approximately 5% of healthy people harbor brain aneurysms, and fortunately, most do not rupture. Early detection of an unruptured aneurysm can be facilitated by certain symptoms that may offer clues to their existence. These include:

- *Localized headaches*

- *A unilaterally dilated pupil*

- *A drooping eyelid*

- *Double vision*

- *Pain above or behind the one eye.*

Discovering an unruptured aneurysm may lead to prophylactic surgical or endovascular (nonsurgical minimally invasive procedure) treatments depending on their size and estimated risk of rupture. Unfortunately, thirty thousand Americans have a ruptured aneurysm every year, and 10% of them will die before they even reach the hospital. If the sudden, severe, unusual headache symptom of aneurysm rupture is not promptly diagnosed and effectively treated, the risk of rebleeding is between 4% and 10% in the first day, and rises to 30% within 1 month. And when a recurrent rupture occurs, up to 50% of patients may die. Table 9 shows the red flag symptoms of headaches.

There are other types of structural blood vessel abnormalities that can cause spontaneous brain hemorrhages. Of these, arteriovenous malformations or AVMs are the best known. An AVM is an abnormal collection of arteries and veins inside the brain. They are present from birth and are occasionally associated with aneurysms Approximately 300,000 Americans are affected by this condition, although in a large number of those affected (~12%), they are incidental findings causing no symptoms at all. AVMs are less lethal than brain aneurysms, although death associated with a ruptured AVM is as high as 15%. The risk of bleeding from an AVM ranges from less than 1% to 35% per year depending on whether it has bled before (higher risk in those that have already bled; sometimes minor bleeding does not produce symptoms and is only detected by special brain scans), its location in the brain (deep brain location confers a higher risk), and the type of drainage blood vessels associated with it (deep drainage confers a higher risk). More common than bleeding as a complication of AVMs are seizures, fleeting strokelike symptoms, and migraine-like headaches. Treatment of an AVM is guided by the location and accessibility of the AVM, the physical condition of the patient, and the estimated bleeding risk. These range from the treatment of epilepsy with medications, surgical resection, endovascular occlusion, and irradiation of the AVM.

Table 9. Red Flag Symptoms of Headaches

Red Flag Symptoms
Headache associated with fever
Sudden "worst headache of my life"[a]
Headache that is new or different in someone with migraines or other known headache disorder

(continued)

Table 9. (*continued*)

Red Flag Symptoms

Headaches associated with sexual activity, exertion, or coughing

Headaches associated with neurological symptoms such as paralysis/weakness in limbs, imbalance or loss of coordination, numbness, vision problems, confusion, drowsiness, or loss of consciousness

Headaches occurring after age 50 in someone without a known headache disorder

Headaches associated with a stiff neck

Headaches associated with nausea and vomiting or sensitivity to light in someone without a known headache disorder such as migraines

Headaches that wake you up in the middle of sleep or new and persistent early morning headaches

[a] *Classic symptom of a stroke caused by a ruptured aneurysm in the brain. Patient and family-friendly information on brain aneurysms can be found at the Brain Aneurysm Foundation, www.bafound.org.*

The Aftermath of Her Life-Threatening Stroke

Life is lived on the edge of death[1]. A drunk driver can hit us while crossing the street, or we can be victims of a violent crime or terrorist attack. We can drown in a flash flood. We can be killed by a freak of nature. And we can experience a deadly stroke.

For so long, Fiona had wrestled with ghosts that heightened her anxiety—invisible ailments that haunted her dreams with their illusion of reality so powerful that she became a hypochondriac. That morning, Fiona had called her primary care doctor with nonspecific complaints: she could not put her finger on it—she just knew there was something wrong, as though she were close to the edge of death. But because of Fiona's history of psychosomatic complaints, her doctor told her that she would be fine and doubled the dose of her antianxiety drug, Xanax. He had had similar telephone calls from Fiona before, all of which were false alarms. He failed to realize that this time was different. Like the boy who cried wolf, it was now too late for Fiona: her demons had found a way to break out of her head and leap into her physical world. Her worst fears were coming true.

Fiona's stroke occurred suddenly while she was watching a soap opera with her girlfriend, whom she had asked to come round that

---

[1] Joseph Campbell, *The Power of Myth* with Bill Moyers. First Edition. New York: Anchor Books, 1991.

morning because she was afraid. When the convulsions began, Fiona was eating a salad that her girlfriend had brought over. Food particles bubbled up from her frothing mouth while her body shook violently. Invisible hands were trying to break Fiona's neck, choking her as she foamed at the mouth, forcing her head rightward until it could no longer turn, her left arm and left leg kicking vigorously, her body jerking, as she tried to escape demons that leapt into her physical world.

In the emergency room, Fiona's initial brain scans revealed a large brain hemorrhage that filled almost half of the right side of her brain, shifting her entire brain tissue to the left, and crushing it against the inner surface of her skull. The pattern of blood on the scans did not suggest a burst aneurysm or bleeding brain tumor. Instead, it resembled a spontaneous hypertensive hemorrhage, where blood vessels deep within the brain succumb to high blood pressures that split open arterial walls. And yet Fiona always took her prescription drugs—she never missed a pill or doctor's appointment. But her doctor did not treat her labile blood pressures aggressively enough:

"You need to manage your stress," he would say.

FIVE HOURS LATER...

Fiona emerged from the cobwebs of lethargy trying to regain her presence of mind. She found herself lying on a strange bed surrounded by bright lights. Suddenly, it happened again. Her left hand began jerking. It was like an alien limb, and she was unable to control it. The terrifying jerks crept up her arm towards her face, which had once again turned the other way. As her mind faded, the jerks spread, consuming her entire body, becoming so violent that she accidentally bit a piece of flesh from her tongue and urinated all over herself.

Fiona slipped in and out of consciousness on the hospital stretcher; she heard people screaming. The neurosurgeon yelled to the nurse to begin the "Mannitol" infusion as they rushed Fiona to the operating room in a frenzied convoy of health-care professionals.

Fortunately, the surgery went well. The procedure performed was called *hemicraniectomy*. Part of Fiona's skull was removed to relieve the dangerous pressure that resulted from the spontaneous bleeding inside her brain, and a large blood clot was sucked out. The neurosurgeon had decided to widen the incision during the operation, remove a large skull bone flap, and keep it in a medical refrigerator until the swelling inside her brain reduced, at which point he planned to suture the bone flap back to its original place on Fiona's skull.

Several days later, in the postoperative intensive care unit, Fiona's eyes flickered open. Her arms were tied down, and a large tube, which carried oxygen into her lungs, protruded from her throat. Infusion bags, each of which was connected to her via long, thin plastic tubing, enshrined her. A large white bandage was wrapped around her head like a turban, through which emerged another tube that drained bloody fluid out of her brain. The radio at the nursing station was playing the Bob Marley classic, "No Woman No Cry," but Fiona did not have the strength to cry—she conserved what was left of it to keep herself alive.

When I looked at Fiona as she lay still on the hospital bed, I did not know what to say or whether she would even understand me. She looked her age—61 years, although when I moved a little closer, the swelling below eyes made her look older. But it was the inner eyes of her soul that made be tremble. They stared right at me, speaking a language I had become familiar with in all my years of doing this.

"Don't let me die . . ."

The fight was not over—the ailments that had haunted Fiona's dreams were all coming true, pushing her closer to the edge of death. All the years of Xanax and false alarms were rehearsals—as though she knew this day was coming.

Fiona developed a high fever. During her convulsions, her salad had gone down her windpipe and had caused a life-threatening pneumonia. When I listened to her chest with my stethoscope, I heard dry crackling sounds all over her lungs, like the noise made by rubbing hair between the fingers close to the ear. Her blood cultures grew a rare bacteria species on the Petri dish that I had never heard of before, which was insensitive to most antibiotics. Within days of her surgery, Fiona had developed sepsis—a whole body inflammatory state in response to widespread infection, which is also known as blood poisoning. Fiona's condition spiralled out of control. And although I tried to save her, pull her from the edge of death, Fiona died on her fifth day in hospital.

Comment

Fiona had a spontaneous (nontraumatic) hemorrhagic stroke (Figure 8 shows an example of a hemorrhagic "wet" stroke as seen on a brain scan). This type of stroke is more fatal than its ischemic counterpart, and while causes of both overlap, the treatment of spontaneous hemorrhagic stroke is different. Unlike ischemic (dry) strokes, which can be treated emergently with thrombolytic therapy (t-PA), no specific drugs have been shown to consistently improve outcomes after hemorrhagic (wet) strokes. Although rigorous scientific evidence is lacking, good theoretical rationale exists for early surgical evacuation in specific cases. In general, individuals with large life-threatening hemorrhages, cerebellar hemorrhages greater than 3 cm in diameter (measured on a brain scan), or hemorrhages resulting in disabling neurological deterioration may benefit from surgical evacuation.

The natural history of stroke is such that approximately 15% of its victims die, 10% end up in long-term care facilities, 40% have moderate-to-severe and persistent disability, 25% have minor impairments, and 10% will experience almost complete recovery. The causes of clinical deterioration after strokes are either directly related to the stroke itself or to its complications. These include extension of the blood clot or thrombus in ischemic (dry) stroke, expansion of the bleeding in hemorrhagic (wet) strokes, swelling within the brain from dying cells, aspiration pneumonia (as in Fiona's case), heart attack related to massive adrenaline surges, heart failure, pulmonary embolism related to a blood clot in the immobile leg, and metabolic disturbances. These complications must be anticipated with prophylactic measures where applicable, and heightened vigilance for early detection and early treatment.

Seizures are abnormal electrical discharges from injured, irritated, or developmentally irregular brain tissue, although the nature of the underlying injury is not always apparent. Seizures are notorious for their visually frightening manifestation of violent body jerking. They typically last less than 2 minutes, but if you're watching someone have one, it can be the longest 2 minutes of your life. Seizures may be complications of brain injury due to ischemic or hemorrhagic stroke or stroke mimics such as brain tumors, brain infections, too low and too high blood sugar levels, or certain drug intoxications.

When strokes are heralded by seizures (as in Fiona's case), an underlying stroke mimic requires more systematic exclusion with the aid of brain scans and certain blood tests. These seizures may occur within 2 weeks of a stroke (early-onset seizures) and beyond 2 weeks, even years after, a stroke has occurred (late-onset seizures). Seizures occurring in the setting of stroke increase the risk for subsequent seizures or poststroke epilepsy—a condition characterized by recurrent and randomly occurring seizures. Seizures complicate approximately 5% of strokes, and they

A] Hemorrhagic "wet" stroke   **B] Normal elderly brain**

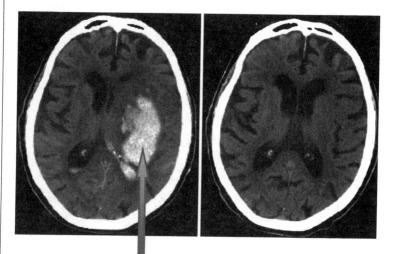

Bleeding inside

the brain (white)

Figure 8. CT (Computer Tomography) Scan showing a hemorrhagic "wet" stroke—a glimpse into the brain

are a common cause of epilepsy in the elderly. Early seizures after stroke are more common after hemorrhagic strokes, although their presence does not predict 30-day fatality. It remains unclear why some patients with strokes develop seizures and others do not. When seizures occur, it is important to lay the person down on his or her side—not on the back, because the tongue can fall backwards and block the airway— and simply wait it out. Do not give the person something to bite down on, like a spoon. Contrary to popular belief, it is not possible to swallow your tongue. Seizures can be effectively controlled with anticonvulsant drugs.

Interlude

According to Herodotus, to have much knowledge but no power is the bitterest pain among men.

Perhaps this is true.

Fiona died. Elizabeth died. Sam and Anna died spiritually. And Omar was left with just one working limb after his second stroke.

There must be a way to empower the public—to assimilate the urgency of stroke and its cardinal symptoms so that more can be saved. To take the lessons learned—the innumerable deaths caused by stroke every year—and transform the bitterest pain.

Sometimes I wish I had a bulletproof soul so that I can withstand my bad days on the hospital wards. In the midst of my wishing, I begin to think about Pedro—his journey of a thousand miles, and his reunion with Lucy. I think of Andrew and remember how a stroke saved his life. I recall the ice cream parlor where he experienced the deepest joy he had ever known. I pictured him sitting there, beaming, and holding a wafer cone with his good right hand.

I look at my watch, it is already 7.30 a.m. Time for morning rounds. I put on my white coat and adjust my tie before heading downstairs to the nurses' station, to begin a new day.

PART TWO

Unusual and Underrecognized Stroke Syndromes: Clinical Manifestations, Causes, and Treatment

Ondine's Curse

Even the Gods are vulnerable to love, for when she laid eyes on him she no longer wanted to be free. Her soul soared through eternity, above the twin peaks of life and death, all she could do was think about him. And then, Ondine, Water Goddess, sacrificed immortality for love.

Palemon was swept off his feet by the winds of Ondine's passion. So captivated was he that he vowed that his "every waking breath would be a testimony of his love and devotion." And it was true that for a time the lovers enjoyed a fairy tale life. But then, inexplicably, Palemon began a secret affair with another woman. The day came when Ondine discovered his betrayal. Exploding in rage, she cursed him, invoking the vow he once made. "Dare to sleep" she screamed, "and you will cease to breathe!"

With one curse, sleep for Palemon became a fatal act. "If I sleep, I die..."[1]

Another fetal loss: three miscarriages in 2 years. Rachel could not take it anymore. It had been 2 years since her marriage to Hugo, since the doctor visits began. They had visited so many fertility experts. They had tried herbalists, acupuncturists, conventional reproductive specialists, even mystics—all to no avail. Instead, countless tests and hormone pills

---

[1] The above story is an adaption by the author from German mythology and the book *Undine* by Friedrich de la Motte Fouque (Hippocrene books: New York, 1990).

brought anger and depression into their lives. The young couple had already begun marriage counseling: they barely touched each other anymore. Then one evening Hugo returned home from work holding two flight tickets in his hand. "Let's get away from it all," he said to her, "let's take a vacation and start over again."

Their chosen destination was a small island by the North Atlantic Ocean not too far from where Ondine, the water goddess, may have roamed. Rachel and Hugo relaxed over the days, rediscovering with joy the playfulness of love. And then one day, after an energetic swim, as Rachel emerged from the water, the large rocks on the beachfront suddenly began oscillating before her eyes. There appeared to be two images of everything on the beach: two Hugos lying on two deck chairs, two cabanas, even two sets of her footprints on the damp sand. But it was the wind on her cheeks that caused her to panic—the intense pins and needles sensation all over her face and inside her mouth that provoked her cry for help—just before she collapsed, and Hugo, seeing her fall, dropped his glass in fear and ran across the grainy white sand to her side. Rachel was having a stroke. She spent 2 days at a local hospital on the main island where she was stabilized. But because specialized stroke care was unavailable, Hugo arranged for an air ambulance to transport his wife back to the United States.

Despite having regained her presence of mind, Rachel's stroke had left her with several problems. She had difficulty swallowing thin liquids and a disabling lack of dexterity. She also maintained an unusual head posture: it was tilted to the right in order to compensate for double vision caused by a stroke-induced misalignment of her eyes. When she arrived at one of the major teaching hospitals where I work, my colleague, who was "on call" that night, evaluated Rachel. He confirmed her stroke with brain scans, and because Rachel was only 29 years old, ordered a special battery of tests designed to detect causes of stroke in young people.

When I took over Rachel's care the following morning, the stroke unit nurses reported to me that Rachel had episodes of progressive loud snoring throughout the night, punctuated by alarming long pauses in her breathing. Hugo had also observed this. He had told the nurses that Rachel's breathing was "scary," that the pauses they had observed occurred whenever she slept, even during daytime naps. The nurses responded to Hugo by reassuring him that his wife most likely suffered from *obstructive sleep apnea*—ubiquitous and treatable sleep disorder common among overweight individuals and characterized by loud snoring and repeated cessation of breathing for 10 seconds or longer during sleep.

But my physical examination on Rachel revealed neurological abnormalities that suggested something different—a more ominous cause of her sleep-disordered breathing. When I reviewed the results of Rachel's tests—sleep studies, cardiac studies, blood tests, and brain scans—my heart sank. Rachel had Ondine's curse. Her "dry" stroke had damaged critical breathing centers in her brain. I identified a bright smudge of dead brain tissue on her brain scans located within a brainstem region called the medulla oblongata. From here traverse pathways descending from automatic breathing control centers. [Automatic breathing is breathing that occurs under unconscious control such as while sleeping.] Rachel had lost automatic breathing function, although her ability to breath voluntarily was preserved. Whenever she tired, her breathing would also tire until it ceased completely. Indeed, those alarming long pauses in her breathing that the nurses observed while she slept were deadly, a sign of imminent respiratory failure. And Rachel's recurrent miscarriages offered clues to the cause of her stroke. The special battery of blood tests revealed evidence of a condition known as antiphospholipid antibody syndrome: a blood clotting disorder, often resulting in unexplained fetal loss. The syndrome can also cause stroke and migraines. Rachel was high risk for death during sleep. Like Palemon, she needed to remain awake or risk death in her dreams.

Grief has a thousand faces, each with unique contours of despair. I remember Rachel's face when I told her what was wrong. I remember Hugo's face, too. And then I thought of Palemon, and I wondered what his face looked like when Ondine cursed him. I thought of life and death and the fragility of health. I thought of love.

We cannot change what has already happened; all we can do is interpret it. Rachel's miscarriages now made sense, but that did not matter anymore. As I explained the diagnosis to Rachel and Hugo, I noticed a change in her face. She looked faint—as if she were about to pass out, overwhelmed by the tragedy of what should have been a happy getaway. I saw her breaths becoming shallower and her eyes begin to fade as I broke the news to her. It must have been the shock of her diagnosis: it had made her light headed, throwing her into a twilight state between sleep and wakefulness, and shutting down her ability to breathe. She needed an emergency breathing tube to prevent suffocation. "Activate the Rapid Response Team!" I instructed the nurse standing beside Hugo, looking right past him—past his contours of despair, past the terror that shaped his face. My focus was on Rachel and the race to keep her alive: she needed a mechanical ventilator to support her breathing.

In one tragic, bewildering moment, their young marriage would be changed forever by a curse from another world. Rachel would likely need the ventilator machine for the rest of her life. And as I inserted the breathing tube down her throat, Hugo stood there: a shell-shocked bystander at the scene of his own tragedy.

Comment

Ondine's curse arises from German mythology, in which the cost of infidelity was a curse that condemned the unfaithful lover to staying awake forever. The loss of automatic breathing prohibits sleep, which depends of automatic breathing. Falling asleep becomes dangerous because patients will cease to breath and suffocate to death.

The dissociation between voluntary and automatic breathing can be explained by selective damage or dysfunction of these breathing pathways as they diverge within the medulla oblongata region of the brainstem (Fig. 9). Fortunately, Ondine's curse is rare. An infantile form also exists. It is a genetically inherited condition that is more common than the adult form, which may be caused by stroke. The treatment of Ondine's curse involves creating an artificial passage in the neck, through which a tube is inserted for lifetime ventilation on a life-support machine, especially during sleep, or in some cases, using a diaphragmatic pace maker.

While Ondine's curse remains rare, sleep-disordered breathing has a strong relationship with stroke. Another disorder called obstructive sleep apnea (OSA)—one of the most common sleep disorders in people—is present in almost 50% of stroke patients. OSA is characterized by turbulent snoring during sleep, between which are interspersed long pauses or silent periods (usually greater than 10 seconds) of breath holding due to upper airway obstruction, followed by loud snorts and body movements that often signify the return of breathing. This temporary cessation of breathing causes a drop in the oxygen concentration in the blood and may lead to sudden irregularities in heart rhythm (cardiac arrhythmia) and surges in blood pressure. As this process continues untreated, the risk of hypertension, heart disease, and stroke grows, while morning headaches and excessive daytime sleepiness become more problematic. OSA can be diagnosed from the information reported by a witness and confirmed with sleep studies (called polysomnography) in a sleep clinic. It is prevalent among overweight or obese individuals and may improve with weight reduction and avoidance of sleeping pills, tranquilizers,

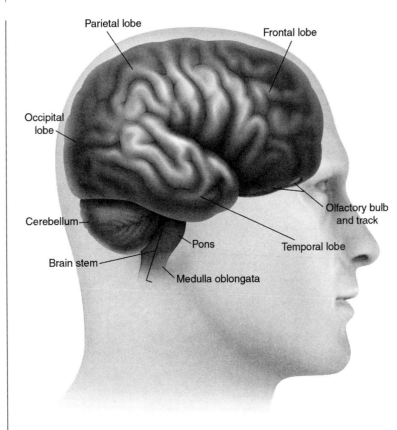

Figure 9. Anatomical regions of the brain

Illustration by Thom Graves, © Thom Graves.

tobacco, and alcohol. In addition to these measures, nasal continuous positive airway pressure (CPAP) should be offered. This treatment not only reduces the risk of stroke but also of heart attack and premature death.

A Stroke that Exiled Her Left Side of Space

Black mascara drew attention to the absence of fear in her eyes, or was it the presence of indifference? Her dark red lipstick appeared skewed, tracing sloping lips around the paralyzed corner of her mouth. There was a stain on her pink blouse—not from the cake she had been slicing when she slumped, but from a laceration above her left eyebrow. And yet Gloria looked indifferent to it all, as if she did not care, blatantly ignoring the signs of stroke on the left side of her body. She had *anosodiaphoria*—a term used to describe a patient's indifference or inability to experience an emotional reaction in response to stroke symptoms.

Gloria had been celebrating when it happened. The stroke gate-crashed her brain damaging centers that were responsible for analyzing space. Her body language was strange, almost paranormal: she appeared to banish the left side of her body, condemning them to exile in the left side of her world. Gloria's *hemineglect* was palpable; she did not even flinch when I sutured the deep cut above her left eyebrow. She did not answer my questions when I stood on her left side. But when I walked around the hospital stretcher to her right side and asked her what was wrong, she responded calmly that she was fine, glancing at me with a bemused smile.

The emergency room was unusually quiet that night. The usual cacophony of beeps and blinking lights from life support machines was absent. Even the overhead paging of crisis management physicians and respiratory therapists was conspicuously missing. But the silence was eerie—as if something bad were about to happen. At that moment, I saw two middle-aged women approaching me. They had long faces and wore identical black dresses as if they were in a funeral procession.

"You must be her family," I said.

The conversation that followed was intense—the kind of dignified intensity where tears are restrained behind a breaking dam of desperate emotions. There is an African proverb that says, "Thunder is not yet rain." Standing there, in front of Gloria's sisters, I saw dark clouds of grief fill up their hearts until there was no space left, and although I did not see it, I could smell the oncoming rain.

Suddenly a loud cough jolted me. Gloria's face was turning pale.

"Oh my God, what's happening to her?!" Gloria's sisters began to panic and cry.

The blood oxygen monitor revealed critically low values and Gloria's heart rate accelerated dangerously. In that moment, two nurses and I began the resuscitation effort. The fight to save life had begun. Gloria's vomit trickled down her windpipe, filling up her lungs with remarkable speed and suffocating her. When I increased the oxygen flow from the machine by her bed and adjusted Gloria's breathing mask, I felt death watching us, listening to the echoes that bounced off the walls—the cries of her sisters in the empty emergency room.

Slowly, the oxygen saturation in Gloria's blood began to rise, and her gasping was replaced by more organized breathing. She was going to survive this episode. And throughout the drama, Gloria's face remained turned to the right side: it never drifted to the left or even to the midline, as if something sinister were there, which she must avoid, and which she alone could see.

Comment

One of the most bizarre manifestations of stroke is hemineglect. It is most frequently caused by damage to the right brain, which is responsible for the perception of space. Conversely, strokes occurring in the left brain may damage language centers and cause an array of abnormalities, which range from nonsensical speech to a total inability to speak (Figure 10 shows functions of the left and right brain hemispheres).

Hemineglect is an inability to recognize one-half of space. It is not "denial" of a hemispace as is often thought—it is an "unconscious inability" to recognize it. And because right-brain injury causes left-sided problems and left-brain injury causes right-sided problems, the left half of space is the side typically affected in this syndrome. Simply put, the left half of space is no longer registered by the right brain. As a result, individuals like Gloria with hemineglect may only eat food on the right side of the plate, they may only groom the right side of their bodies (bathing, shaving, dressing), and they may only respond to interaction in their right visual field.

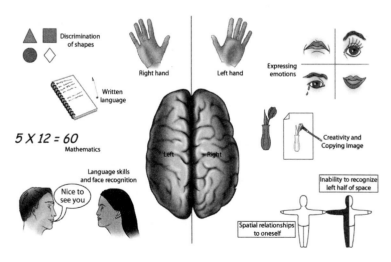

Figure 10. Major functions of the left and right brain hemispheres
Illustration by Thom Graves, © Thom Graves.

These individuals may not hear sound that originates on the left side (even though sound travels pretty fast to the right), they may not recognize their left arm or leg, and they may not register painful stimuli applied to the left limbs even when sensory nerves are working. Moreover, during visual search, these individuals may fail to cross the midline of space to the left, causing them to read only the right portion of a sentence or only appreciate the right half of a picture.

The disability from this syndrome is profound. It is associated with a poor outcome on key functional activities. Nevertheless, partial recovery can occur during the first few days after the stroke, but complete recovery is less common.

As effective drug treatments continue to be investigated with limited success, behavioral therapy has become the mainstay of treatment for hemineglect. The goal is to improve the individual's ability to explore the neglected space. Frequent reminders of the existence of neglected limbs and space can be facilitated through touch and interaction, and individuals should be encouraged to turn their heads from right to left during scanning. In addition, self-alerting devices may help, but it is most important to educate caregivers and encourage them to monitor and manipulate the environment of individuals with hemineglect by placing functional items on the right, and making sure that the environment is safe.

An Unknown White Male Who Could Only Blink His Eyes

I looked at him and guessed he was in his late 30's or early 40's. He appeared well groomed with perfectly manicured toenails. His eyes were fixed in midposition, and I observed a rare blink or two. There was something familiar about him, as though I was having a déjà vu. The nurse told me that he hadn't moved since he arrived on the critical care unit. He didn't grimace or flinch during the numerous body-piercing procedures. The Unknown White Male was vegetative—or so I was told. Despite being awake, he did not respond to any form of internal or external stimuli, including pain. His brain scan showed a nondisplaced skull fracture with a small underlying blood clot, which did not appear sufficient to explain the severity of his neurological condition. As I looked harder, I saw a dark area in a region of the brain called the pons. Unknown White Male had had a stroke: I speculated that it must have been caused by trauma and dissection of an artery at the back of his neck from the presumed robbery assault. The location of this stroke could cause his head-to-toe paralysis, and the trauma to his head may have caused shearing of his neural networks that could explain his vegetative appearance. But there was still something missing, which I could not explain. It was in his eyes. Though fixed in a forward gaze, they seemed alive.

I introduced myself to him as is customary even before a comatose patient, and asked if he was in pain. At that point a colleague walked over to the bedside and told me not to bother, insisting audibly that it was a futile exercise. I felt an eerie déjà vu. I asked for a Spanish interpreter and was told that they had tried that already. Then I asked for a French interpreter.

What happened next still stands alone in my mind.

"Est-ce que vous avez la douleur?" I asked, "Est-ce que ça vous fait mal?"

Everyone was stunned—even the life-support machines went silent. Tears began to roll down Unknown White Male's face. It was the first sign of outer awareness.

Through the French interpreter, I was able to get him to move his eyes up and down but not horizontally. He could also blink to my command. Every other movement was paralyzed and he could no longer feel touch, temperature, or pain. But by codifying his blinks with a yes or no, I used the alphabet and a multiple-choice format in French to complete the interview. His name was Didier.

Comment

Locked-in syndrome has been described as "the closest thing to being buried alive."

It is a most devastating form of stroke. In this condition, an area of brain called the pons (see Fig. 9) is damaged by stroke, and all voluntary muscles throughout the body, except certain eye muscles (blinking and vertical eye movements) are paralyzed. As a result, locked-in individuals cannot speak or move, but they can think and reason—they are fully cognizant of the world around them. In The Count of Monte Cristo Alexander Dumas vividly depicted a character that was "a corpse with living eyes." But one of the most powerful descriptions of locked-in syndrome was by one of its victims—a Parisian journalist Jean-Dominique Bauby, who dictated one of the most extraordinary books ever written, The Diving Bell and the Butterfly, by blinking to indicate each individual letter of an alphabet.

Didier's stroke was caused by dissection of an artery that supplies the brainstem. Dissection refers to a tear in the wall of an artery often due to trauma, including chiropractic manipulation of the neck, but also during minor strains such as the rare cases caused by extension of the neck at a beauty parlor while getting your hair done. Dissection may also be caused by cocaine ingestion, and it can occur spontaneously. When caused by nontraumatic events, dissection is sometimes treated with blood thinners such as warfarin, to prevent progression of stroke.

Sadly, there is no specific treatment for locked-in syndrome; focus of treatment is on nursing care, rehabilitation therapy, and prevention of recurrent stroke. However, just like other forms of non-traumatic "dry" strokes, thrombolytic therapy with t-PA may significantly reduce disability when given within 3 hours of symptom onset.

A Stroke that Turned Him Into a Living Statue

For weeks he had been imprisoned in isolation. And then one morning, after another night of impossible sleep, he had had enough. He went to the bathroom, opened the cabinet, and emptied the entire bottle of painkillers into the granite mortar he used to mix his shaving paste. He ground the pills into a talcum residue and dissolved the powder in drops of tap water. With a used syringe, he drew the solution into the needle. Mumbling Sade's name and looking up, he saw a disheveled stranger in the mirror: a primitive man with severely chapped lips protruding through a dirty black beard. The man's eyes were desperate. Ladi continued to stare at the face in the mirror trying to find a reason not to go through with it, trying to convince himself that she would come back and their lives would return to normal. But he couldn't find a reason to stop. A hand carrying a syringe inched towards a large pulsating vein in the bearded man's neck. He did not flinch until the injection was complete. And then Ladi fell the ground.

I do not presume to know all of the things that man desires. But I have treated some of the things that man does not desire: loneliness, sickness, and a slow protracted and agonizing existence. Herodotus tells us, "When life is so burdensome, death becomes a sought-after refuge."

The psychiatric emergency room can be a haunting place. Some patients hovered by the nursing station talking to invisible people, while others lay on hospital stretchers staring into space. And though Ladi's face was in front of me, I could not really see him, as if he were hiding behind a strange mask. I thought, however, that he could see me. There was a hypervigilance about him, like a wax portrait at Madame Tussauds. His eyes roamed, staring at nothing. He remained immobile, verbally inert, and indifferent to pain. Ladi was akinetic and mute—the needle had pierced the carotid artery in his neck and caused a stroke. Small particles of the crushed painkillers had clogged arteries that carried blood to his frontal lobes. This was why I was called. The psychiatrist asked me to transfer Ladi to my unit because there was nothing more he could do.

The following day, when I walked into Ladi's room, I saw a young lady sitting in a chair.

"Can he hear me?" she asked.

Sade was by his bed. The cleaning lady who found Ladi on the bathroom floor had called her.

"He can hear you," I said.

Six weeks had lapsed since that nightmarish day, and Sade, his lost and now found Sade, never left his side. She never stopped talking to Ladi or reading him stories. And though he did not move, he could still look at her: though he could not smile, he could still shed tears. I treated him with different stimulant drugs and drugs that increased the dopamine levels in his brain. Everyday he was bathed and groomed, and fed through a stomach feeding tube. Multiple times, he was turned around to prevent bedsores. He received range-of-motion exercises. For several hours a day, he was propped up in an armchair by the window, and through it all he did not move, through it all Sade remained at his side, praying and reading, and then praying some more.

And then one morning, as she read to him, she felt his hand move. "Is this really happening?" His hand moved again, and Sade burst into tears.

There is nothing more dramatic than a theater of human suffering, and there is no greater victory than the triumph of the human spirit. If indeed miracles exist, then I was witnessing one that morning as Ladi emerged from a tomb of akinetic mutism. It was hospital day 43. As I approached his bedside during my evening rounds, I heard him whispering his first words to her.

"I am sorry."

Comment

Akinetic mutism (akinesia means loss of movement) has also been called "coma vigil." It is characterized by a state of physical inertia and quiet vigilance despite preserved nerve pathways responsible for movement (motor) and sensation. Patients are awake and immobile and appear unresponsive to external stimuli (including pain), except for visual following. Akinetic mutism should be distinguished from "locked-in syndrome," which can result from damage to the pons (Episode 9). Strokes that cause akinetic mutism injure the medial frontal lobes on both sides of the brain. These regions are critical for programming, initiating, and executing movements. Information related to external stimuli, internally generated movements, and motivation converge in these brain regions, where they are processed before being transferred to motor centers for execution. In addition to akinesia and mutism, bilateral strokes affecting the medial frontal lobes of both brain hemispheres may cause paralysis restricted to the legs that resembles spinal cord paralysis.

Man in a Barrel

Organ failures—heart, kidney, and one time, even respiratory failure, had dogged Rupert's journey up to this moment. But now, aged 65, for the first time in his life, he felt whole. He felt complete. Happiness was no longer out of his reach, confined to vacation spots in his dreams. It was real.

Rupert was doing the washing up, whistling his favorite tunes, when he experienced a sudden discomfort, a crushing sensation inside his chest. It was as if his heart were being squeezed from the outside. He began sweating profusely and hyperventilating. Within seconds he had stopped moving—frozen between fight and flight. The saucer in his hand fell to the ground. He had been here before. From the shadow lands of bad dreams, the fear stalking him had finally broken in. The next scene was familiar to him. Confronted with the imminent danger, his heart quaked, trying to burst from his chest, trying to escape a fatal arrest. When the choking began, it was too late to call out his wife's name. He fell to the ground. A loud crash, then a long silence. He gagged once more before becoming motionless on the kitchen floor.

THE DREAM ...

Rupert stood alone in the middle of an open space unable to move his arms and upper body. It was as though they were trapped inside an invisible barrel. He did not know how he got to this strange place or why he could not move his arms and upper body, but he was not afraid. To anyone looking, the indifference on his face would appear unnatural. In search of answers, he began flipping through the pages of memory. He wanted to find out how he had become trapped inside an invisible barrel. He wanted to know where he was, how he got to this strange place. He turned the page of memory overleaf, but it was blank. Subsequent chapters were filled with meaningless pages written in vanishing ink. Only the page numbers were visible. After sometime he stumbled across a group of bold letters. It was a name. Then he saw her face. It was the most beautiful face he had ever known. She was standing in an empty room next to a soda machine and was wearing a black dress. Was she weeping? Rupert wanted to touch her grief as he continued to read, but he could not move his arms and upper body.

The next pages were blanks—blank after blank until suddenly countless italic letters appeared in long rows; row upon row of exclamations broken only by a set quotation marks around a capitalized noun. The noun was STROKE. He read this word with a pounding heart. It pounded hard, slowing down only when her face appeared again. Her eyes were blood red. Had she been crying?

More words followed but in couplets as though he had double vision and sentences were skewed. They seemed to be heading towards a spiral of more words in the middle of the page. Feeling dizzy, he tripped. Only then did he realize that he was the man lying on the page, that his beloved was kneeling over him, trying to lift him up from the floor.

An ambulance worker in a black jacket with "EMT" written on the back appeared on the next page immediately after the words over which he had tripped and fallen. They spelled "too late". This was the last page.

. . . .

Aristotle believed that dreams could reveal to physicians early changes in the body not perceptible during the day. He implied that our dreams possess an uncanny capacity to reach through time, beyond waking life, and grasp its content from the future.

When Rupert woke up from his dream, he found himself in an unknown place and on a strange bed. It looked like a hospital room. He did not know how he got there. Something was terribly wrong. He could not move his arms and upper body. It was as though he were trapped in an invisible barrel. His nightmare had followed him into the real world. He looked around the hospital room unable to move his arms and upper body and was consumed with fear. The indifference in his dream was replaced by real panic. Only his head and his legs could move. When he turned his head, he saw her walk into the room, wearing the same black dress that she wore in his dream, looking straight at him with tears in her eyes. It was his wife. But unlike before, these were not sad tears: they were joyful tears adorning the most beautiful face he had ever known.

"I thought you weren't coming back," she said. "After you collapsed in the kitchen and the ambulance brought you here, the doctors said it was too late. They said you'd had a cardiac arrest, that you weren't coming back."

It is true that I said this. Even though Rupert had beaten the odds so many times before, it is true that I did not think he would survive this episode. I did not think he would regain meaningful function of his brain. He had all the poor prognostic signs for recovery: resuscitation began late—at least 30 minutes following his collapse at home, and when the ambulance crew arrived and found him without a pulse, it took another 40 minutes of CPR (cardiopulmonary resuscitation) before he regained a normal heart rhythm. But what convinced me the most that Rupert would not make it was not the large "border zone" strokes on his brain scans, it was the paucity and quality of brain responses during my neurological examination on his third hospital day.

Sometimes there is no greater relief than being wrong. There is no greater glory than when the human spirit defies scientific evidence in a fight for survival. And there is no better teacher for us doctors on the frontline.

Rupert's surprising recovery was nutrition for my soul. It reminded me that modern medicine deals with odds and not absolutes, and that the end of certainty is the beginning of opportunity for our dreams to come true.

When I entered the room, I did not know what to say or how much emotion to display. I walked over to Rupert's bedside, next to where his wife was sitting, and placed my hand on Rupert's hand. With my other hand, I reached for his wife's hand, pausing for a moment as she dried her tears, before applying a gentle squeeze.

Comment

The overall survival following an out-of-hospital cardiac arrest is dismal—less than 5%. One of the complications in survivors is a stroke syndrome called "man-in-the-barrel." This syndrome is used to describe a patient who can move both legs spontaneously or in response to pain but is unable to move his or her arms as if the arms and upper body are trapped in a barrel. Most cases occur in those who suffer sustained drops in blood pressure or circulatory failure that is severe enough to cause coma. After Rupert collapsed in his kitchen from a cardiac arrest, he suffered sudden low blood flow to his brain (called hypoperfusion), which damaged vulnerable "border zone" areas where delicate blood flow exists between major cerebral arteries. Unlike the more common strokes due to blood vessel blockage by blood clots, these dry strokes are due to sudden hypoperfusion. Certain border zone regions in the brain contain fibers responsible for moving the arms and upper body, which explains, in part, why they are paralyzed, and the legs and face are spared. Due to the nature of its underlying causes such as cardiac arrest or circulatory shock from massive blood loss or widespread infection, most patients with man-in-the-barrel syndrome die, although some like Rupert survive and may go on to recover arm strength.

The Circle of Dementia

There is something extraordinary about a circle. Of all the shapes in the universe, the circle is the most magnificent. There is something curious, paradoxical in its simplicity.

Imagine playing with a baby: the way he or she grasps your hand and does not know how or when to let go. The way babies babble incoherently or scream out of the blue. Torrential tears are interspersed with giggles and slumber in a circle of parenting. From emotional incontinence to urinary incontinence, these bundles of joy can sometimes test the love of exhausted caregivers.

But there is more than one circle in life. There is the circle of a human cycle where babies develop into adults and adults regress into infancy. Primitive reflexes that babies display such as the grasp reflex disappear during maturation of a baby's brain. And when brains age, the effects of silent strokes can cause these primitive reflexes to reappear on a tragic stage of vascular cognitive disorder (VCD).

Silent strokes are not silent—this is a misnomer. They kill neurons and supporting brain cells indiscriminately, leaving behind a subtle trail of dead tissue, which can be detected by brain scans. They are called "silent" solely because they do not cause obvious stroke symptoms. Indeed, a single attack may have no notable clinical significance—but over time, recurrent assaults may lead to a non-linear time course of cognitive dysfunction.

An old man begins to cry without provocation as a childlike lability returns in life's sequel. His excuses are initially plausible but they soon stop making sense. Defensive behavior surfaces and belligerence is around the corner. He used to be gregarious but now he is reclusive; he used to be stoic but now he is emotional. Visual-spatial dysfunction leads to frequent wandering and getting lost, as his cognitive metamorphosis transforms joy into despair.

Then I start to think of a circle again, only now the circle is filled with familiar faces—fading faces. And like the startling hallucination of a blind man, I think I see my face among them. I think I see my aged face hanging on a branch of my family tree.

Comment

Silent strokes occur in 11 million Americans (4% of the U.S. population) every year. They are a far cry from voiceless. This misnomer was born at a time when we did not know how deadly these "silent" brain attacks were: we thought that they only damaged "functionless" brain cells, which explained why they did not cause classic stroke symptoms, such as sudden numbness or weakness, sudden dizziness, incoordination or loss of balance, sudden difficulty speaking or confusion, sudden blindness in one or both eyes, and sudden thunderclap headache. Clinical studies have shown otherwise: these silent strokes may lead to vascular cognitive disorders (VCD) and a form of dementia that is second only to Alzheimer's disease, although the two may coexist. And because vascular lesions in the brain may coexist with Alzheimer's disease, and because epidemiological studies have suggested that risk factors for vascular disease and stroke are associated with and may intensify the severity of Alzheimer's disease, the definition of vascular dementia has been fraught with controversy, and at the time this book was written, no validated pathological criteria for the diagnosis of vascular dementia is available.

Dementia in any form is a debilitating condition for the patient and a despairing existence for his or her caregiver—so much so that one study found that one-third of primary caregivers of a person with dementia experience depression.

A recent term added to stroke nomenclature is "whispering stroke." Whispering strokes are tiny fragments of classic stroke symptoms that often go undetected. These vehement whispers, so often ignored by doctors and patients, may be associated with decreased mental functioning. The symptoms of whispering strokes are usually so fleeting that conventional brain scans are unable to prove that they were ever even there, and they rarely make the grade required for classification as a TIA (transient ischemic attack, or ministroke). Prevention of silent and whispering strokes can be accomplished by controlling medical stroke risk factors (Table 5) and maintaining a healthy lifestyle.

Interlude

I found a rose at the center of my soul—the one Omar told me to look for. After days of watching it, I noticed that it always turned towards the light, tracking the sun as it moved across my inner being. When night fell, it continued to face the east, waiting patiently for the sun to rise again.

And the sun always rises. Daylight follows even the darkest night. The buttercups in the fields know this; their diurnal motion is linked to the sun in a heliotropic cycle of life like the rose at the center of my soul.

As I sat in my office, I began thinking about Rachel, and Gloria, Ladi, Rupert, and Didier. What they all had in common were strange stroke syndromes, where mystery murders took place in their brains. Rachel had Ondine's curse, Gloria did not recognize the left side of her body, Ladi was a living statue, Rupert was trapped in an invisible barrel, and Didier was like a "corpse with living eyes."

I met each of them during the darkest hour of their night; I watched as their minds buried millions of coffins, each a single neuron, deep inside their brains. I did not tell them that the sun would rise again because I did not know if it would.

But now I have found the center of my soul. I can see the distance from myself—from my periphery. I remember the words of Osho: *The moment you have a center, the periphery can be abused, but not you.*

Perhaps this is the reason for Omar's strength.

I place my stethoscope in my black bag and take off my white coat. On the way out, I stop and look up at the diplomas on my wall. I realize that there is so much they did not teach me, so much they did not prepare me for.

PART THREE

Psychosocial and Physical Challenges After Stroke

Sex After Stroke

Imagine being consumed by the fear of sex—the dread of having another stroke at the peak of pleasure. Imagine flurries of uncontrolled spasms in paralyzed limbs, with each pelvic thrust. Imagine dryness and pain or a urinary accident occurring during sex. Imagine a French kiss— then imagine drooling from a pool of saliva because one cannot clear his or her own secretions from the back of the throat. Imagine the shame of a frail or failed erection. Imagine a life of lost desire or not being able to articulate desire. Imagine the paranoia of hurting him or her. Imagine not being able to feel the caress of a loved one because the sensory nerves of the body suddenly died. Imagine an overnight demise of self-esteem.

We have limbic needs. Every single one of us. We must never dismiss the need for emotional intimacy in stroke survivors or their spouses. I have seen stroke sever intimacy—that space within which two souls commune; I have watched it rip holes in love. In hospital waiting rooms, I have heard the silent screams of unmet limbic needs.

For some stroke survivors, this is a fate worse than death, a punishment that makes them wish they had not survived. But it doesn't have to be this way ...

Comment

There is a great dearth of available information on sex after stroke, and yet for some, this may be one of the most difficult aspects of recovery. It is difficult for both the stroke survivor and his or her spouse or partner. The physical changes that occur after a stroke can adversely affect sexuality, while the emotional changes might arrest it altogether.

When self-esteem crashes, buried in the rubble can be found our libido, our confidence, and our desires. These are replaced by depression, embarrassment, anxiety, and repressed feelings. And while stroke can cause real physical impediments to sexual activity such as vaginal dryness, erectile dysfunction, impotence, loss of movement and sensation, urinary incontinence, and the presence of a urinary catheter, strategies exist for minimizing or overcoming them.

It is important to address the paralyzing fear of sex after stroke. Apart from strokes caused by brain aneurysmal ruptures (Episode 5), recurrent strokes occurring during sexual intercourse are extremely rare, although it is important to seek counsel from medical professionals for any concerns related to resumption of sex.

Most stroke survivors can safely resume sexual activity. Indeed, countless babies have been born by stroke survivors. Their sexual journey may be tough, but it is one that usually ends in triumph. One that demands creative positions in order to minimize pain and optimize penetration, and one that may require specific strategies such as using generous amounts of lubricant jelly or taping a urinary catheter tubing to the side during sexual activity. This sexual journey is often one of exploration, requiring sufficient time, where the search for areas of heightened sensitivity in a body that has been harmed by sensory loss is patiently undertaken. And for those survivors without sexual partners, masturbation remains a safe alternative.

Strokes do not usually cause erectile dysfunction, even when half of one's body is paralyzed. The nerves on the unaffected side are sufficient for achieving and maintaining erections. The greatest obstacle to sex after stroke is fear, and the failure to communicate these fears or ask for help. Additional information on sex after stroke can be found in the American Heart Association's sex-after-stroke guide: Our Guide to Intimacy After Stroke. The National Stroke Association's Recovery After Stroke: Redefining Sexuality is also a useful resource.

The Terror of Crossing the Street

Francis had become isolated and socially withdrawn. Despite successfully completing his speech therapy program and regaining his ability to complete sentences, Francis did not want to talk to anyone; he wanted to be left alone. His new fear was more paralyzing than the stroke he had suffered. There were nightmares: impending peril in recurrent dreams. Every night he would wake up trembling just before he was run over by an oncoming car. The horror of his phobia made him irrational. The more control of his limbs he gained, the more afraid he became—especially today. The time had come for him to go outdoors—to make the dreaded journey and traverse the haunting few yards of the pedestrian crossing on his way to his doctor's appointment.

When the trucks came to a halt, his heart began to thump. The pounding grew louder when he saw the haste in the headlights before him. Images of his recent fall collided in his mind like a fatal accident. It was as though Francis had suffered two simultaneous strokes—one psychological and one physical, both feeding off his fear. His gait had regressed back to a form that resembled a baby trying to walk—which made him stagger and sway like a drunkard. His broad-based stance, ostensibly a swagger, was a poor attempt to compensate for his axial instability. And despite his cane, which acted as a fulcrum, each stride was awkward and stiff due to his reluctance to flex his knees during leg swings.

As his fear reached crescendo, Francis was jolted by a young man who almost knocked him off balance before disappearing across the street with his iPod. He had, with some trouble, regained his footing when a child appeared beside him and asked if he was all right. He nodded, reassuring her with a smile, before casting his eyes back across the pedestrian crossing.

There was something different about today—a positive feeling in the air. Today he would push back the handicap that made him fall repeatedly: he would rise up against fear, determined to live free, intent on getting to the other side of the road.

When the traffic lights turned red and the pedestrian light changed to "walk," Francis began his odyssey across the busy intersection. He was lunging from his pelvis, his legs widening with each lunge—a caricature of a stride, a step—each one elicited with a sigh of relief. He concentrated on maintaining his center of gravity as his trunk swayed back and forth around his cane. He focused on his feet, watching his heavy heel strikes on the concrete slabs. The faulty communication between his limbs and his brain forced him to depend on his eyes. He had never come this far before. He had crossed the midway point of his journey, and the pedestrian lights were still not flashing. As he approached the other side of the road, his heart quickened, engines revved, and a song of victory burst from his heart. For more than 6 months, Francis had failed to cross the street before the lights changed back. And now he had done it. He stood on the sidewalk, night falling around him. He felt as though he could fly. For the first time since his stroke, he felt free.

Comment

The recovery from a damaged brain begins in the heart. It begins with a grieving process, which we need to understand. An acute state of anguish typically follows a period of shock, denial, and disbelief, before anger and fruitless bargaining with the deity ends in mourning and acceptance of the new reality. But there is a fine line between the normal grief that accompanies bereavement, and major depression. Indeed, when suicidal thoughts accompany intense feelings of hopelessness, profound changes in appetite and prominent sleep dysfunction, major depression needs to be considered and appropriate treatment instituted. In Francis's case, the excellent recovery of his ability to communicate (Table 10 shows tips for language recovery after stroke) was eclipsed by the psychological trauma of his recurrent falls. This disability from his stroke led to an irrational fear of open spaces (agoraphobia) that plagued his dreams and caused depression.

Post-stroke depression is common. Approximately 37% of stroke survivors develop depression, and up to 22% may be diagnosed with major depression. Post-stroke anxiety disorders are also common and often co-exist with depression. The majority of cases of post-stroke anxiety disorders are agoraphobia. Agoraphobics usually do not leave the "safe zone" of their home. The reasons for this are myriad, and in Francis's case, were reinforced by a fear of falling. Reports indicate that more than one-third of stroke survivors experience falls during the first year after having a stroke due to problems related to walking, and of those who fall, more than one-third require medical treatment (Table 11 categorizes walking problems and offers guidelines for recovery). Agoraphobics are plagued by dread of public or unfamiliar places where escape would be difficult. Exposure to these situations may trigger a panic attack. Cognitive behavior therapy (CBT) and/or specific drugs may help this disorder. Table 12 shows the symptoms and signs of depression.

Table 10. Tips for Language Recovery After Stroke

Speech Therapy Tips

Language relearning can be very frustrating for stroke survivors. Patience and positive reinforcement of successfully completed tasks are important for confidence building.

With guidance from speech pathologists, family and caregivers should practice speech therapy concepts being addressed with stroke survivors.

The two major categories of language abnormalities (aphasias) diagnosed by medical professionals are fluent (receptive) and nonfluent (expressive) aphasias. In expressive (nonfluent) aphasia, comprehension of speech is generally preserved (which is why individuals with this form of aphasia are easily frustrated and often depressed), although stroke survivors have significant word-finding difficulties and loss of grammatical markers such as coordinating conjunctions and prepositions (telegraphic speech). These individuals also have problems naming (speech may be filled with "paraphasic" errors, which may be phonemic paraphasias such as substituting "ladder" for "letter" or semantic paraphasias such as substituting "table" for "chair"), and problems reading and writing. Interestingly, individuals with expressive (nonfluent) aphasia retain their ability to sing familiar songs—an asset that is exploited in melodic intonation therapy, which superimposes melodic and rhythmic patterns into everyday utterances as an initial step. Family and caregivers can augment formal speech therapy programs by slowing down their rate of speech, exercising patience and allowing ample time for responses, using concrete yes/no choices to facilitate an accurate response, and not continuously correcting the stroke survivor's speech.

Treatment of fluent (receptive) aphasia is often hinged on the presence of some comprehension. In the absence of comprehension, these individuals rarely benefit from formal speech therapy programs.

Help for stroke survivors with aphasia can be found at the National Aphasia Association, www.aphasia.org.

Table 11. General Guidelines to Aid Safe Recovery of Walking After Stroke

General Tips for Walking Again

A damaged brain retains a capacity to reorganize itself and use different regions to get a specific task accomplished. This functional reorganization may be positively and negatively influenced by patterns of use or disuse respectively, such as repetitive training versus non-use of a limb that has been affected by stroke.

Meaningful and attainable goals should be set at outset. Encouragement is key.

It is important to practice exercises independently of structured physical therapy programs and avoid long inactive periods. Family and caregivers may help with these activities.

The best exercises are those that emulate the function of the activity that has been lost (task-specific practice).

Mental practice/rehearsals also activate brain networks and are more effective than no practice, especially in those with more severe impairments.

Be patient: even a healthy child's brain takes approximately 1 year to learn to walk. Relearning to walk after stroke takes time in adults: minor physical gains are quantum leaps in the brain.

Use prescribed walking aids and orthotic devices.

Stretching and bending exercises should be performed every day to prevent stiffness and painful joint contractures.

Falls should be reported to your doctor (they may be more serious than they appear to an untrained eye).

A good exercise program should involve educating family members and caregivers and include written information with illustrations.

It is important to create an environment for stroke survivors that is stimulating, is devoid of constraints (trip hazards), and encourages social interaction in the real world.

Table 12. How to Recognize Depression in Stroke Survivors or Caregivers

Symptoms and Signs of Depression

Feeling hopeless or helpless
Loss of interest in normal daily activities
Crying spells without an obvious reason
Loss of energy and fatigue
Significant weight gain or weight loss associated with appetite
   changes
Poor sleep or oversleeping
Restlessness, irritability, and trouble concentrating
Suicidal thoughts or behavior
Loss of libido

The Accommodador—A Caregiver's Point of Giving up

I clean him, wash him, I brush his curly hair. I change his clothes, feed him, exercise him, struggle to get him onto the wheelchair. I wheel him to the balcony, read to him, heave him back onto the bed. And then I turn him in the middle of the night to prevent bedsores. Once in a while we go to the park. I push his wheelchair to the baseball field and watch the young kids play and the pigeons fly away. Once in a while, I think he can see me, I think he can hear me, but the experts say I am wrong—they say that I am a ghost to him, and these fragments of his inner awareness are figments of my imagination. So I gave up my imagination along with its figments. Sometimes I want to be like him—to live without senses in the wilderness of my mind.

The sun and moon have been pulled out of my soul. I feel there is no night or day: no sky, no clouds, no rain, and no wind—just emptiness, a vast open space. Everything is gone. There are no voices here: no whispers, no laughter, no crying. The music has gone away. I feel as if a great loss has displaced everything that I own.

It took me a while to get here—to arrive at the "acomodador." Five years has lapsed since the stroke stole him from me after 30 years of being together. Now that I am here, and I still cannot find him, I don't know what to do. Perhaps this is the worst kind of suffering—not knowing what to do. I wish I were still traveling—still hoping. There is nothing here for me: no feeling, no sleep, and no dreams. I am hollow. I am cold. I am a caregiver with no one to hold.

Comment

The road to "acomodador" —the point of giving up—is a lonely one for the caregiver.

In his book, The Zahir[1], Paulo Coehlo describes the "acomodador", an ancient practice in North Mexico, as an event in our lives that is responsible for us failing to move on: a trauma, a bitter defeat, a disappointment in love, and in this case, a stroke in a loved one. In order to progress beyond the "acomodador," we must first recognize it and then free ourselves from that point of giving up, so that we are left with the instincts that develop out of the various difficulties and tragedies we have experienced.

Caregiver's depression is a national crisis. In fact, one study found that 33% of caregivers of stroke survivors experienced depression, which was higher than the depression rate of the stroke survivors themselves. Caregivers' depression has been linked to the stroke survivors' disability, their depression, their level of social activities, and caregiver employment status. The challenge of caregiving can be daunting. The reality can overwhelm even the strongest among us. The needs of stroke survivors can be innumerable. There are physical needs, which include bathing, dressing, grooming, diaper changing, transferring from bed to chair and back, shopping for groceries, preparing meals, giving medications, and managing finances. There are emotional needs, which include cognitive dysfunction, denial, loss of ability, agitation, mood swings, social withdrawal, social stigma, panic, sexual response changes, and even psychotic behavior. And through it all, caregivers remain the number one cheerleader, the lover and companion, the therapist, the secretary, the nurse, the bookkeeper, and the housekeeper. In the face of these challenges, it is not surprising that caregiver depression is common. It is most important for the caregiver to seek care for any symptoms of depression or anxiety or difficulty coping. Once identified, these problems can be effectively treated with drugs or psychological therapy, including caregiver support group therapy. Tables 13 and 14 listsome helpful tips and resources for caregivers.

---

[1] Paulo Coelho, *The Zahir*. New York: Harper Perennial, 2005.

Table 13. Tips for Caregivers

Caregiver Tips
Understand your loved one's goals and work with your medical team to achieve attainable goals.
Do not neglect your own health such as missing your own doctor's appointments, forgetting to take your own pills, not exercising, and not eating a healthy diet.
Remember that you are not "superhuman." Learn to ask for help or say "yes" to offers of help. You must take breaks from caregiving.
Remember to seek professional help if you have difficulty coping. The gulf between difficulty coping and major depression is not the great distance some think it is.

Table 14. Resources for Caregivers

Online Resources for Caregivers
National Stroke Association online support programs for stroke families in partnership with "lotsa helping hands": www.stroke.org. This is a web-based caregiving service that allows families, friends, and neighbors to create a community to assist a family caregiver with daily activities.
National Family Caregivers Association: www.nfcares.org.
American Heart Association forums for stroke survivors and family caregivers: www.strokeassociation.org.
Stroke Survivor: www.strokesurvivor.com. Resources for stroke survivors and their caregivers.

Interlude

A great adversary resides within our minds. It is our imagination—a place of great power, where logic can be overthrown by a matrix of mad thoughts, so daring they sometimes invade reality.

A patient once told me that a dead man was happier than he was. He added that if he had the choice between life and death, he would choose neither. Instead, he continued, "I would rather be unborn."

Rudyard Kipling said, "If you can force your heart and nerve and sinew to serve your turn long after they are gone and so hold on when there is nothing in you except 'will' … yours is the earth and everything that is in it." It is our "will," Kipling says, that "can meet with triumph and disaster and treat these two imposters just the same."

Some people never find the "will" to go on, like the caregiver who had reached her giving-up point. But others do. When Francis crossed the street that day, he overcame a great adversary and freed himself back into the world.

I have learned that stroke is a journey for survivors and their families. It begins on a lonely road—on a difficult journey to the center of the soul. But if we make it there, if we find our "will," then we, too, can overcome great adversaries and be freed back into life, into all the good and bad that is in it.

PART FOUR

Recovery from Severe Stroke

Abiku: Breaking the Curse of Childhood Death

In the mythology of the Yoruba tribe of Nigeria, royal ancestors are reincarnated as forces of nature or Orisha—gods of the earth. Shango is the fourth king of the Oyo kingdom, a legendary warrior with magical powers. The day he died, the sky was darkened by a great storm, and a bolt of lightning cleaved the heavens in two. Thunder shook the earth, and village hamlets burst into flames. That night, Shango returned as the god of thunder and lightning.

Oshun was the youngest and prettiest of his three wives. Deified as a river goddess and known for her ability to promote childbirth and cure infertility, Oshun also had the power to protect children from *Abiku*—the curse of childhood death.

With its gentle twists and turns that flow southward into the Atlantic, the fresh water of the Oshun River symbolizes the sensuality of Oshun's beauty. Every year, she drew hundreds of barren women to her muddy riverbanks, where they would offer prayers and sacrifices to her in a bathing ritual. These women sought the *gift of Oshun*—a baptism of fertility by the river goddess.

The cowskin mat which Seriki had spread on the damp soil was covered in her footprints. She had just slipped on a white linen garment after bathing in the river. Still dripping with fresh water, she began dancing barefoot by the Ayan tree. There, on the banks of the Oshun River, Seriki danced all night in the ancient fertility ritual, invoking the spirits of her ancestors, dancing into an invisible world, approaching a trance state. The necklace of blue beads which hung around her neck jangled to the rhythm of her gyrating hips. She raised her arms above her head, displaying the brass bracelets on her wrists, which slid down her arms as she danced feverishly, making her offering to the river goddess. She was about to be condemned by the village elders for blocking the stream of human life, and this was her last chance to receive the gift of Oshun.

The ascent of the sun between the peaks of the Yoruba hills intensified her incantation. Seriki's chanting grew louder and louder until she began to scream at the top of her voice. There was an overwhelming upheaval in her gut. Her soul burst from her bosom and soared into the sky to commune with the gods. An explosion of thunder followed with giant streaks of lightning piercing the loud sound like a sword. Shango had awoken. His fiery temper ignited by Seriki's intrusion caused the Oshun River to swirl and overflow her banks.

THIRTEEN MONTHS LATER ...

I was in Africa, in a remote outpost clinic at the end of a winding dirt road, a few miles from the Oshun River, and thousands of miles away from New York City. The makeshift clinic served a local village inside a sacred forest whose inhabitants worshiped Shango. We were in the treatment room, one of two rooms in the clinic. The place was dilapidated and unclean. A dysfunctional ceiling fan creaked in the dry heat. Windows jammed open between torn mosquito nets let flies in, in droves. They fed on patients who were too weak to object. I was visiting a colleague, posted to the clinic as part of his national service. What the clinic lacked in basic medical supplies paled in comparison to the unfathomable events I am about to narrate.

It was as though the world had stopped turning—a still frame within which the baby's jerks seemed to last forever. The jerks were so violent they dislocated his shoulders. All I could see were the white of his eyes. His pupils had rolled upwards and backwards within his eye sockets, as if they were searching frantically for something buried deep within his head to make the fitting stop. When the baby stopped seizing, I noticed that his left face was drooping and his left arm and left leg were not moving. They were flaccid and paretic, raising the likelihood of a pediatric stroke masking itself as epilepsy. I noticed three tribal scars on both of the baby's shoulders. (My colleague later told me that the baby had been marked with the sign of Abiku—so that he would be recognized if and when he was reborn.) Closer inspection of the child's body revealed that the bottoms of his feet were badly burned. I had treated burn victims in the past, but I had not seen anything like this. The perfect symmetry of the burns on the soles of the baby's feet raised the monstrous spectacle of child abuse, and the clinical constellation of signs was as perplexing as it was horrific. My colleague saw the shock on my face and politely asked the baby's mother to leave the room.

My colleague told me the story of an evil spirit in Yoruba mythology called "Abiku" (*abi* means "give birth," *iku* means "death"). Abiku is a demon with no stomach that preys on newborn children. It has no physical form, only a smoky image, which prowls through villages with an insatiable appetite for young souls. One manifestation of Abiku is childhood seizures. The local cure for these seizures involves an ancient ritual. The exorcism takes place in a cave, deep within the sacred forest where medicine men would hold down an Abiku child and burn his or her feet repeatedly with fire in an attempt to drive out the demon. The mother must deliver the child to village elders on the night of the ritual and return to her hut, where she waits until the child is returned. She believes that the medicine men will save her child. She is not different from most mothers who will do anything to save their child.

I walked over to the clinic window and saw Seriki waiting a few yards from the entrance. She was oblivious to the rain and the lightning bolt that struck the nearby beehive. She was dancing wildly, invoking the spirit of her ancestors, speaking the language of Orisha, dancing in a trance until her breath and blood became one. The medicine men had failed to save him, and now the fate of her child was in the hands of Orisha.

There is an African proverb that says, "When the heart overflows, it comes out through the mouth." So it was with the force of a breaking dam that Seriki's heart burst open, its contents gushing through her mouth in a loud cry, so loud we did not hear the thunderstorm outside or the sound of rain on the tin roof over our heads. We heard only Seriki crying out her child's name.

"Durosinmi, Durosinmi, Durosinmi." (The name means, "Stay and bury me.")

Some people believe that the cause of suffering is human craving. They believe that the end of suffering is linked to our ability to transcend our deepest desires and live free of attachment. I believe that human craving cannot be separated from human life.

"Durosinmi, stay and bury me," repeated Seriki before doubling over from the visceral agony in her womb.

"Take me instead," she pleaded in vain to the gods of nature. Durosinmi was waking up. I looked down at the baby, my heart filling with pain. In his innocent eyes was a heart-breaking fear as he hyperventilated in the small cot in front of us. Suddenly, he tried to scream—but the guttural sounds from his weak and slurry cry could not gain traction. The child was consumed by terror. He must have thought that we were medicine men returning to burn his feet.

Seriki ran into the treatment room soaked in rainwater. She scooped up the child from inside the small cot and cradled him against her breast until he stopped crying. She sang to him in a beautiful soft voice until he drifted to sleep in her arms. I saw the painful saga in her eyes, full of love and death. Perhaps it was the fear in her eyes that I mistook for death—or perhaps it was her tears—the streams of human life that had ended in miscarriages, before her son was born.

The sun rolled off the dome of sky. Darkness began to fill the earth. A car pulled up in front of the clinic entrance sounding its horn. It was time for me to leave. I had to return to Oshogbo, the large town 200 miles away. When we reached the end of the winding dirt road at the foot of the Yoruba hills, I told the driver to stop for a moment so that I could look back one last time. The sunset cast a golden blanket over the sacred forest.

I said a silent prayer for the child and then told the driver to move on. The hills became smaller and smaller, finally disappearing from sight.

9 MONTHS LATER ...

The rainy season is over and the river is calm. The gentle ripple of fresh water along the banks of the Oshun River form a harmony with the little boy's laughter, sprinkling the air. Seriki chased her toddler around the Ayan tree in a game of hide and seek. It is a new season in her soul. The beauty of the landscape is brightened—infinitely—by the smile of her healthy, living son.

Durosinmi has recovered completely from his stroke. He runs around in circles, almost knocking over the pottery bowl filled with white stones from the riverbed, placed on a cowskin mat by the tree. Seriki is wearing a long white gown adorned with jewels and yellow copper. The brass bracelets on her wrists jangle as she chases her son across the grass. By the Oshun river, they play, hearts overflowing with joy which spills from their mouths.

Comment

The signs of stroke in babies are different from those in adults. Specific clues include:

- *Delays in developmental milestones such as walking or talking*

- *Favoring one side of the body or early handedness (children usually do not develop handedness until after 1 year)*

- *Visual recognition difficulties*

- *Fainting episodes. Seizures are a common manifestation of stroke in babies, as depicted in the story of Seriki. Some estimates suggest that stroke accounts for up to 10% of cases of infant seizures.*

The first few days before and after birth are a high-risk period for baby strokes. In fact, the stroke rate in infants rivals that of the elderly in the first month of life. Recent estimates put this rate at 1:4,000 births, which is much higher than in older children. Maternal trauma, maternal cocaine use, certain congenital infections (like parvovirus B19), congenital heart disorders, maternal blood clotting disorders, pre-eclampsia, and a variety of genetic disorders, have all been implicated as causes of baby strokes.

The good news is that up to 40% of these babies (like Durosinmi) recover fully—even after large strokes. Others are left with long-term neurological problems, especially cerebral palsy (an umbrella term for neurological disorders that appear in infancy and early childhood, associated with developmental or physical disabilities that don't worsen over time), cognitive impairment, and epilepsy.

There is no proven role for clot busters such as t-PA for the treatment of "dry" strokes in babies. However, anecdotal cases of "wet" strokes successfully treated with surgical evacuation of large hemorrhagic clots have been reported, and the placement of "shunts" into the fluid cavities of the brain to drain dangerous accumulation of blood or prevent swelling of the fluid cavities in the brain (hydrocephalus) may also be performed.

Though frightening to observe, these babies are not defenseless against stroke. They are not unprepared. They possess an uncanny ability to withstand the invasion of their brains despite the lack of evidence-based treatment options in this age group. Their tiny brains, which are more "plastic" than yours and mine, can skillfully reroute neural networks around damaged areas, recruiting neighboring cells to replace fallen neurons in the fight for life.

The Lazarus Phenomenon: A Miraculous Outcome after Stroke

The audition before the gods was a spoken word symphony of a thousand voices—an *a capella* of prayer in perfect unison. The acoustic energy in the sanctuary was palpable, and the stained glass windows, hallowed by Christian saints, reverberated with the sound of the Nicene Creed. The pews were packed with bowed heads of men and women in black, chanting memorized verses over and over again. Behind the raised altar was a large choir whose members were draped in blue velvet robes, seeming to flow into the sea of black outfits. There was a closed coffin in front of the white podium, adorned with a gold-plated cross. The coffin was enshrined by a mini-garden of white carnations, gladiolas, and dagger fern arranged in casket sprays. Periodically, loud cries would pierce through the rhythm of voices and then fade as quickly as they came. With the growing decibel of wailing, I wondered where the threshold stood for God to hear their pain. There were tears on many faces: visible and invisible tears, seeping through worn-out hearts and pooling on the rusty bunkers that sheltered weary souls. And then there was Paul. When the congregation became silent, Paul slipped out of the front row pew and walked towards the white podium to give the eulogy for Harry.

Rumor has it that Paul's father, who was also his mother's pimp, murdered her over a 20-dollar tip she had received from a client, and then killed himself. Since the age of 15, Paul had lived on the streets of Harlem doing whatever he could to survive, except for crime. He ran errands for the old and disabled, collected tin cans from garbage piles and bagged them for recycling, washed cars for strangers for whatever fee they were willing to pay, and cleared construction debris for illegal contractors almost every day. When night fell, Paul would retreat to a shed by the railway tracks, made with black dustbin liners and abandoned clothing, and held up by cardboard boxes and empty crates. There he would lie, invisible to passersby, listening to the music of trains going by. There he would dream of Harlem Day—an annual celebration of health and heritage—the day when he and his mother would laugh and play.

After Paul's mother was killed, and his father had been found dead on the scene, the young boy had run away and had begun living on the streets. But Harry, who always paid attention to the missing children flyers, had found him. His timing could not have been more perfect. He rescued Paul from the terror of nonentity and freed him with his acts of loving. Harry pulled Paul from the edge of a mental cliff and gave him hope. Over subsequent years, Harry and his wife Vicky restored Paul. They turned him into a fine young man.

Paul stood at the pulpit looking down at his handwritten notes, almost losing control of his emotions. Collecting his thoughts, he crumpled up the piece of paper in front of him and slid it into his trouser pocket. Taking a deep breath, he looked up at the many that had gathered before focusing on Vicky.

I was at the funeral that day to honor Harry—a leader among a coalition of community health advocates that I co-chaired. Three other people had been killed on the day Harry died, although the newspaper article the following morning barely mentioned their names. The headline in the Harlem Gazette read, "Drunk driver slays local health champion." The hit-and-run driver, later apprehended by the police after crashing into a fire hydrant, was found drunk in a Buick littered with empty bottles of vodka.

Harry was a man of few words, but when he spoke, the wisdom of his words could resonate for days. I once heard him say to Paul, shortly after he had taken the young boy in, that there is no better teacher in life than adversity.

Harry and his wife Vicky were one of a kind. What most would call coincidence, they saw as signs—even obvious things like the brightness of stars when the moon is not full.

When I looked at Paul, standing in the pulpit, he was staring at Vicky. I watched him looking at her, the silence that separated his tears from his opening words unsettling the funeral crowd.

"Harry was a good man," he began. "He gave so much to so many people, especially those he did not know and would likely never see again. Harry was a humble man. He once told me that he often wondered whether he deserved to be a giver. He told me that there are many who have nothing to give—not even a smile: those fighting to stay alive in the midst of advanced disease. These are the folks for whom he fought and died: those who have nothing to give up but life itself."

In the middle of the eulogy, commotion in the crowd interrupted Paul: a loud cry, then sudden disorder was coming from Vicky's pew. Paul ran to the scene, jumping off the raised altar, knocking over the flowers that enshrined Harry's coffin. In an instant, the house of prayer had become home of pandemonium. Vicky! But I couldn't see through the crowd that swarmed her. I heard panic, cries, and the frantic calls for a doctor. The scene possessed the texture of a bad dream. I stood in disbelief among the crowd. Then the enormity of the shock brought me back to reality.

Love does not end with death: it is not buried with our bones. Even though our limbs decompose to become one with the earth, the love in our soul remains until the end of time. Today felt like the end of time.

I had to push my way through the thick crowd that had gathered around Vicky's pew. When I got to her side, two doctors were already there, trying to save her: two strangers trying to save the life of another stranger in the midst of a thousand strangers. Vicky could barely speak as she dangled on the church pew. Slurred words drooled out of her drooping mouth. Her right arm and right leg were flaccid, her head and neck appeared forcefully deviated to the left side, and her eyes were like cavernous pits from which fear streamed forth.

"Call 911," I said to the stranger behind me, "tell them someone has had a stroke."

It took 15 minutes for the ambulance to arrive. It felt like eternity. During this time, the great sorrow that filled the air inside the sanctuary began to dissipate. The choir had started singing the Lord's Prayer. Soon, the entire congregation joined in, singing in harmony as Paul wept on his knees and I grappled with the surreal tragedy unfolding before me.

A taxi took me to the hospital. I got out near it, consciously slowing my stride as I approached the building. Then a strange calm came over me. I looked up at the sky noticing the stars shining brightly and the crescent moon. I wanted to believe that this was a sign and not coincidence. I wanted the stars to be angels clothed in light approaching the earth from all corners of the universe to witness a miracle about to take place in our world.

Paul was inconsolable. Images from his former life flashed in his mind. He saw his mother's face—her black and blue eyes beneath the bleeding brow. He saw his father's fists shatter her front teeth as he beat her to death over a 20-dollar tip. He saw himself running into the night as fast as he could, from the wrath of a madman. Then he watched himself go mad; he saw his body squatting in a shed by the railway tracks as sounds of trains went by. He saw the faces of the old and disabled he had run errands for. The old and disabled who gave him food. Then he saw Vicky and Harry—felt their loving deep in his soul—he rejected all thoughts of Vicky's death.

It was 9.45 p.m. The doctors and nurses had been working on her for more than an hour. I asked the neurologist whom I was meeting for the first time, what Vicky's brain scans had revealed.

"They were normal, doctor," he said.

I struggled to maintain my grip on hope.

This was not a "wet stroke" since bleeding in the brain is detected instantly by scans. Vicky was having a "dry stroke": it does not usually appear on brain scans in its earliest stages, during the gasping phase, when brain cells are deprived of oxygen. In dry strokes, brain scans usually become abnormal during the dying phase of brain cells, when their death is imminent or has just occurred. Vicky still had time left—approximately 1 hour and 15 minutes. She still had time for t-PA.

The chaos in the emergency room was subsumed into an atmosphere of war on hospital stretchers. The sound of life support machines and defibrillator shocks on the chest of strangers became the sound of the clashes between life and death.

Vicky appeared lifeless, although she was awake. The cavernous pits that were her eyes had now emptied all their fear; her limbs crashed down onto the stretcher when the neurologist raised her right arm.

By now t-PA was flowing through her veins from a thin plastic tube connected to an inverted vial hanging on a steel pole. I knew firsthand that in the presence of such a large stroke, t-PA's effect is sometimes muted, even though the chance of recovery is greatly improved.

Some of us believe in signs and not in coincidences. The bright stars were angels clothed in light gathering to witness a miracle in our world.

The miracle is called the "Lazarus effect." When Vicky rose from the hospital stretcher, I did not know whether to laugh or cry or sigh. Paul ran to Vicky's side. I watched their embrace. From Heaven, Harry gazed upon the sanctity of Vicky's recovery.

Comment

Increasing numbers of observers are witnessing rapid and often complete resolution of stroke symptoms within 24 hours of treatment with t-PA. This dramatic phenomenon known as the "Lazarus effect" is defined scientifically as at least 50% reduction in disability at 24 hours after treatment, as measured by the National Institute of Health Stroke Scale (a clinical scale used to assess stroke severity). Figure 11 shows time-dependent changes, which appear on brain scans during an ischemic "dry" stroke, in the presence and absence of a Lazarus effect.

In specialized stroke centers, newer but more invasive stroke treatments are gaining momentum. These offer the advantage of an extended treatment window from 3 hours to 6 hours or 8 hours from the onset of stroke symptoms. They include intra-arterial (directly into the artery unlike more traditional but indirect intravenous/vein route) administration of thrombolytic drugs directly into offending blood clots inside the brain, and the use of mechanical clot-extracting devices that are navigated through an artery in the groin all the way to the blocked artery in the brain!

The Lazarus effect appears to be more common after intra-arterial administration of t-PA. Although not formally approved by the FDA (at the time this book was written) for the treatment of acute stroke, intra-arterial thrombolysis with t-PA has gained widespread acceptance among stroke experts. Another intra-arterial treatment available for stroke patients is the use of the MERCI (mechanical embolus removal in cerebral ischemia) retriever. This corkscrew-shaped device, approved by the FDA, can remove clots from clogged arteries in the brain within 30 minutes. Intra-arterial treatments offer some advantages over intravenous administration of t-PA, including an extended treatment time window from 3 hours to 8 hours. The major disadvantage of intra-arterial treatments is their limited availability (often restricted to large academic stroke centers) due to the need for advanced technology and highly specialized personnel.

At the 2007 International Stroke Conference of the American Stroke Association in San Francisco, researchers from Ohio State University tried

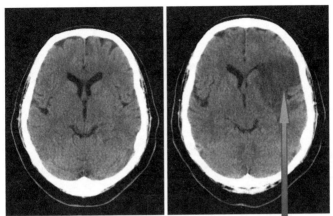

Normal Brain

Ischemic "Dry" Stroke

Dark region represents
dead brain tissue (infarction) in a "dry"
stroke. [This finding is usually not
seen on a CT scan during the first 3
hours from the onset of stroke
symptoms, and may never appear if
blood flow is quickly restored and a
Lazarus effect occurs]

Figure 11. Computed Tomography (CT) scans of the brain showing an Ischemic "Dry" Stroke

to determine which factors led to the Lazarus effect. In their group of 108 stroke patients treated with intra-arterial clot busters, almost 25% of patients experienced the Lazarus effect. The most important predictor was time to treatment: the earlier patients arrived within the treatment window, the greater the chances for dramatic improvement. This is yet another reason why we must not hesitate to call 911 when stroke is suspected and get our loved ones to the hospital in time.

EPILOGUE

It is the end of another long day. The vision of Themis, the blind-folded goddess holding up her scales, has vanished from my windowpane. She was a Titan, daughter of the union between Earth and Sky, who ruled long before Zeus was born.

I hang my white coat on a hook behind my clinic door wondering why the goddess is blind. Is it because our eyes are windows that allow illusions to distort our hearts? Is it because we need to lose sight of ourselves in order to gain insight into the needs of others? Perhaps we must be blind so that we do not judge the strangers that lie on our hospital beds.

Our patients are made up of more than their past and more than their present. They are made up of more than the risk factors of yesterday and the symptoms of today. They are a part of all of us, woven by the same thread of humanity that holds together the great tapestry of human life. Their cause is our calling: an oath that we swore to uphold, written by Hippocrates in the days of Apollo centuries ago: "We will apply for the benefit of the sick all measures required, avoiding those twin traps of over-treatment and therapeutic nihilism; we will remember that there is art to medicine as well as science, and that warmth, sympathy, and understanding outweigh the surgeon's knife or the chemist's drug … that this awesome responsibility must be faced with great humbleness and awareness of our own frailty."

I walk out of the room remembering all the patients whose stories I have told—those who died and those who survived. Even though their faces come from many different places, they all wanted the same thing—to be relieved of sickness and suffering.

I close the door behind me, recalling the words of Kahlil Gibran—"the wind speaks not more sweetly to the giant oaks than to the least of all the blades of grass, and he alone is great who turns the voice of the wind into a song made sweeter by his own loving."

General References

Caplan, L. R. *Stroke*. St. Paul, MN: AAN Press. New York: Demos Medical Publishing, 2005.

Hutton, C. *After a Stroke: 300 Tips for Making Life Easier*. New York: Demos Medical Publishing, 2005.

Hutton, C., Caplan, L. R. *Striking Back at Stroke: A Doctor-Patient Journal*. Washington, DC: Dana Press, 2003.

Shimberg, E. F. *Strokes. What Families Should Know*. New York: Ballantine Books, 1990.

Prologue

Gordon J. Medical humanities: To cure sometimes, to relieve often, to comfort always. *Med. J. Aust.* 182, no. 1 (2005): 5–8.

Episode 1

American Heart Association. *2008 Heart Disease and Stroke Update*. Dallas, TX: American Heart Association, 2008.

Eggers, A. E. A chronic dysfunctional stress response can cause stroke by stimulating platelet activation, migraine, and hypertension. *Med. Hypotheses* 65, no. 3 (2005): 542–545.

Elkind, M. S. et al. Moderate alcohol consumption reduces risk of ischemic stroke: The Northern Manhattan Study. *Stroke* 37, no. 1 (January 2006): 13–19.

Fung, T. et al. Mediterranean diet and incidence of and mortality from coronary heart disease and stroke in women. *Circulation* 119, no. 8 (2009): 1093–1100.

Glymour, M. et al. Spousal smoking and incidence of first stroke: The Health and Retirement Study. Am. J. Prev. Med. 35, no. 3 (2008): 245–248.

Green, D. M. et al. Serum potassium levels and dietary potassium intake as risk factors for stroke. *Neurology* 59 (2002): 314–320.

Iso, H. et al. Intake of fish and omega-3-fatty acids and risk of stroke in women. *JAMA* 285, no. 3 (2001): 304–312.

Pell, J. et al. Smoke-free legislation and hospitalizations for acute coronary syndrome. *N. Engl. J. Med.* 359, no. 5 (July 31, 2008): 482–491.

Surtees, P. et al. Adaptation to social adversity is associated with stroke incidence. *Stroke* 38, no. 5 (May 2007): 1447–1453.

Wells, A. J. Passive smoking as a cause of heart disease. *J. Am. Coll. Cardiol.* 24 (1994): 546–554.

Surtees, P. et al. Psychological distress, major depressive disorder, and risk of stroke. *Neurology* 70 (2008): 788–794.

Wolf, P. A. et al. Cigarette smoking as a risk factor for stroke. The Framingham Study. *JAMA* 259 (1988): 1025–1029.

Yaggi, H. K. et al. Obstructive sleep apnea as a risk factor for stroke and death. *N. Engl. J. Med.* 353, no. 19 (November 10, 2005): 2034–2041.

Episode 2

Feinberg, W. M. et al. Guidelines on the management of transient ischemic attacks. From the ad hoc committee on guidelines on the management of transient ischemic attacks of the stroke council of the American Heart Association. *Stroke* 25, no. 6 (1994): 1320–1335.

Johnston, S. C. et al. Diagnosis of TIA short-term prognosis after emergency department. *JAMA* 284, no. 22 (2000): 2901–2906.

National Stroke Association Steps Against Recurrent Stroke (STARS). http://www.stroke.org/site/PageServer?pagename=RECUR

Rothwell, P. M. et al. A simple score (ABCD) to identify individuals at high early risk of stroke after a transient ischemic attack. *Lancet* 366 (2006): 29–36.

Sacco, R. et al. Guidelines for prevention of stroke in patients with ischemic stroke or transient ischemic attack: A statement for healthcare professionals from the American Heart Association/American Stroke Association Council on Stroke: Co-sponsored by the Council on Cardiovascular Radiology and Intervention: The American Academy of Neurology affirms the value of this guideline. *Stroke* 37, no. 2, (February 2006): 577–617.

Tayal, A. H. et al. Atrial fibrillation detected by mobile cardiac outpatient telemetry in cryptogenic stroke. *Neurology* 71 (2008): 1696–1701.

Trends in Intake of Energy and Macronutrients, United States, 1971–2000. *Morbidity Mortality Weekly Report*, 53, no. 4 (February 6, 2004): 80–82.

Episode 3

Adams, R. et al. Recommendations for improving the quality of care through stroke centers and systems: An examination of stroke centers identification options: Multidisciplinary consensus recommendations from the Advisory Working Group on Stroke Center Identification Options of the American Stroke Association. *Stroke* 33 (2002): e1–e7.

Brott, T., and Bogousslavsky, J. Treatment of acute ischemic stroke. *N. Engl. J. Med.* 343, no. 10 (September 7, 2000): 710–722.

CDC. Prehospital and hospital delays after stroke onset – United States, 2005–2006. *MMWR Morb. Mortal. Wkly. Rep.* 56, no. 19 (May 18, 2007): 474–478.

Douglas, V. C. et al. Do the Brain Attack Coalition's criteria for stroke centers improve care for ischemic stroke? *Neurology* 64, no. 3 (February 8, 2005): 422–427.

Evenson, K. R. et al. Prehospital and in-hospital delays in acute stroke care. *Neuroepidemiology* 20 (2001): 65–76.

Gillum, L. A., and Johnston, S. C. Characteristics of academic medical centers and ischemic stroke outcomes. *Stroke* 32 (2001): 2137–2142.

Greenlund, K. J. et al. Low public recognition of major stroke symptoms. *Am. J. Prev. Med.;* 25, no. 4 (November 2003): 315–319.

Gropen, T. I. et al. Quality improvement in acute stroke: The New York State Stroke Center Designation Project. *Neurology* 67, no. 1 (July 11, 2006): 88–93.

Hacke, W. et al. Thrombolysis with alteplase 3 – 4.5 hours after acute ischemic stroke. *N. Engl. J. Med.* 359 (2008): 1317–1329.

Morgenstern, L. B. et al. Increasing public recognition and rapid response to stroke. *A National Institute of Neurological Disorders and Stroke Symposium: Improving the Chain of Recovery for Acute Stroke in Your Community.* Bethesda, MD: National Institutes of Health, Department of Health and Human Services, Office of Communications and Public Liaison, National Institute of Neurological Disorders and Stroke, National Institutes of Health, Department of Health and Human Services, 2003:1–9.

National Institute of Neurological Disorders and Stroke rt-PA Stroke Study Group. *N. Engl. J. Med.* 333 (1995): 1581–1587.

Schneider, A. et al. Trends in community knowledge of the warning signs and risk factors for stroke. *JAMA* 289 (2003): 343–346.

Williams, L. et al. Stroke patients' knowledge of stroke: Influence on time to presentation. *Stroke* 28, no. 5 (1997): 912–915.

Williams, O., Noble, J. M. "Hip-hop" stroke: A stroke educational program for elementary school children living in a high-risk community. *Stroke* 39, no. 10 (October 2008): 2809–2816.

Episode 4

Brust, J. C. M. *Neurological Aspects of Substance Abuse.* 2nd Edition. Boston: 2004.

National Institute on Drug Abuse, "Monitoring the Future" Survey 2007. http://www.drugabuse.gov/infofacts/cocaine.html

Williams, O., Noble, J.M., Brust, and J.C.M. Stroke associated with cocaine abuse: No longer just a problem of the young. *Neurology* 66, no. 5 (March 2006, Suppl. 2): A384.

Episode 5

Eldow, J., and Caplan, L. Avoiding pitfalls in the diagnosis of Subarachnoid hemorrhage. *N. Engl. J. Med.* 342 (2000): 29–36.

Kissela, B. M. et al. Subarachnoid hemorrhage: A preventable disease with a heritable component. *Stroke* 33, no. 5 (May 2002): 1321–1326.

Kowalski, R. et al. Initial misdiagnosis and outcome after subarachnoid hemorrhage. *JAMA* 291 (February 18, 2004): 866–869.

Naidech, A. et al. Predictors and impact of aneurysm rebleeding after subarachnoid hemorrhage. *Arch. Neurol.* 62 (2005): 410–416.

Schievink, W. I. et al. Sudden death from aneurismal subarachnoid hemorrhage. *Neurology* 45, no. 5 (May 1995): 871–874.

Stapf, C. et al. Predictors of hemorrhage in patients with untreated arteriovenous malformation. *Neurology* 66 (2006): 1350–1355.

Episode 6

CDC. Prevalence of disabilities and associated health conditions among adults—United States, 1999. *MMWR* 50 (2001): 120–125.

Fewel, M. E. et al. Spontaneous intracerebral hemorrhage: A review. *Neurosurg. Focus* 15, no. 4 (October 15, 2003): E1.

Labovitz, D. L. et al. Prevalence and predictors of early seizure and status epilepticus after first stroke. *Neurology* 57 (2001): 200–206.

Episode 7

Ali, L., and Avidan, A. Sleep-disordered breathing and stroke. *Rev. Neurol. Dis.* 5, no. 4 (2008): 191–198.

Ali, A., and Flageole, H. Diaphragmatic pacing for the treatment of congenital central alveolar hypoventilation syndrome. *J. Pediatr. Surg.* 43, no. 5 (May 2008): 792–796.

Nannapaneni, R. et al. Retracing "Ondine's curse." *Neurosurgery* 57, no. 2 (August 2005): 354–363.

Episode 8

Parton, A. et al. Hemispatial neglect. *Journal of Neurology Neurosurgery and Psychiatry* 75 (2004):13–21.

Episode 9

Jean-Dominique Bauby. *The Diving Bell and the Butterfly: A Memoir of Life in Death.* Paris: Editions Robert Laffont, S.A., 1997.

Alexandra Dumas, *The Count of Monte Cristo.* Barnes and Noble Classics series. New York: Spark Educational Publishing, 2004.

Smith, E., and Delargy, M. Locked-in syndrome. *BMJ* 330 (February 2005): 406–409.

Episode 10

Combarros, O. et al. Akinetic mutism from frontal lobe damage responding to levodopa. *J. Neurol.* 247, no. 7 (July 2000): 568–569E.

Nagaratnam, N. et al. Akinetic mutism following stroke. *J. Clin. Neurosci.* 11, no. 1 (January 2004): 25–30.

Yang, C. P. et al. Diminution of basal ganglia dopaminergic function may play an important role in the generation of akinetic mutism in a patient with anterior cerebral arterial infarct. *Clin. Neurol. Neurosurg.* 109, no. 7 (September 2007): 602–606.

Episode 11

Nichol, G. et al. Regional variation in out-of-hospital cardiac arrest incidence and outcome. *JAMA* 300, no. 12 (2008): 1423–1431.

Sage, J., and Van Uitert, R. Man-in-the-barrel syndrome. *Neurology* 36 (1986): 1102.

Episode 12

Covinsky, K. et al. Patient and caregiver characteristics associated with depression in caregivers of patients with dementia. *J. Gen. Intern. Med.* 18, no. 12 (December 2003): 1006–1014.

Gorelick, P., and Bowler, J. Advances in vascular cognitive impairment 2007. *Stroke* 39 (2008): 279–282.

Howard, G., et al. Stroke symptoms in individuals reporting no prior stroke or transient ischemic attack are associated with a decrease in indices of mental and physical functioning. *Stroke* 38, no. 9 (September 2007): 2446–2452.

Jellinger, K. The pathology of "vascular dementia": A critical update. *J. Alzheimer's Dis.* 14, no. 1 (2008): 107–123.

Leary, M. C., and Saver, J. L. Annual incidence of first silent stroke in the United States: A preliminary estimate. *Cerebrovasc. Dis.* 16, no. 3 (2003): 280–285.

Vermeer, S. E. et al. Silent brain infarcts and the risk of dementia and cognitive decline. *N. Engl. J. Med.* 348, no. 13 (March 27, 2003): 1215–1222.

Episode 13

Recovery After Stroke: Redefining Sexuality. http://www.intimaterider.com/images/NSAFactSheet_Sexuality.pdf

Episode 14

Benson, F. et al. *Aphasia: A Clinical Perspective.* New York: Oxford University Press, 1996.

Burvill, P. W. et al. Anxiety disorders after stroke: Results from the Perth Community Stroke Study. *Br. J. Psychiatry* 166, no. 3 (March 1995): 328–332.

Carr, J. and Shepherd, R. *Stroke Rehabilitation: Guidelines for Exercise Training to Optimize Motor Skill.* Oxford: Butterworth Heinemann (Elsevier), 2003.

Helm-Estabrooks, N. et al. *Approaches to the Treatment of Aphasia.* San Diego, CA: Singular Publishing, 1998.

Kelley-Hayes, M. et al. The influence of gender and age on disability following ischemic stroke: The Framingham study. *J. Stroke Cerebrovasc. Dis.* 12 (2003): 119–126.

Ngaire Kerse et al. Falls after stroke. Results from the Auckland Regional Community Stroke (ARCOS) Study, 2002 to 2003. *Stroke* 39 (2008): 1890–1893.

Robinson, R. et al. Escitalopram and problem-solving therapy for prevention of poststroke depression: A randomized controlled trial. *JAMA* 299 (2008): 2391–2400.

Episode 15

Berg, A. et al. Depression among caregivers of stroke survivors. *Stroke* 36, no. 3 (March 2005): 639–643.

Episode 16

Lynch, J. K. et al. Report of the National Institute of Neurological Disorders and Stroke workshop on perinatal and childhood stroke. *Pediatrics* 109 (2002): 116–123.

Mackay, M. T., and Gordon, A. Stroke in children. *Aust. Fam. Physician* 36, no. 11 (2007): 896–902.

Roach, S. et al. Management of stroke in infants and children. AHA Scientific statement. *Stroke* 39 (2008): 2644–2691.

Episode 17

Brott, T., and Bogousslavsky, J. Treatment of acute ischemic stroke. *N. Engl. J. Med.* 343, no. 10 (September 7, 2000): 710–722.

Christofordis, G. et al. Factors associated with a "Lazarus phenomenon" 24 hours following intra-arterial thrombolytic treatment in acute ischemic stroke. *Stroke* 38, no. 2 (2007): 507–508.

Furlan, A. et al. Intra-arterial prourokinase for acute ischemic stroke. The PROACT II study: A randomized controlled trial. Prolyse in acute cerebral thromboembolism. *JAMA* 282 (1999): 2003–2011.

Gillum, L. A., and Johnston, S. C. Characteristics of academic medical centers and ischemic stroke outcomes. *Stroke* 32 (2001): 2137–2142.

Smith, W. S. et al. Mechanical thrombectomy for acute ischemic stroke: Final results of the Multi MERCI trial. *Stroke* 39, no. 4 (April 2008): 1205–1212.

INDEX

Note: Page numbers followed by "*f*" and "*t*" indicate figures and tables, respectively.

ABOUT THE AUTHOR

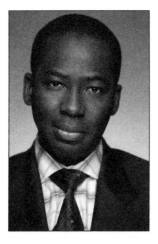

Dr. Olajide Williams is a general neurologist with special interest in stroke. He received his medical degree from the University of Lagos, Nigeria, in 1994. In 1997, Dr. Williams did an internship in internal medicine at Harlem Hospital Center, New York, followed by residency training at Columbia Presbyterian Medical Center (1998–2001), where he also completed his fellowship training (2001–2002). In August 2002, he was made Assistant Professor of Clinical Neurology at the College of Physicians and Surgeons of Columbia University. In May 2004, he completed his Masters degree in Biostatistics from the Mailman School of Public Health at Columbia University through a Patient Oriented Research scholarship provided by the National Institutes of Health. Dr. Williams is board certified in neurology and electrodiagnosis, and practices medicine at New York Presbyterian Hospital (Columbia campus) and Harlem Hospital Center. He is Founder and Director of the Harlem Hospital Stroke Initiative and the Hip Hop Public Health Education Center at Harlem Hospital.

Dr. Williams is a fellow of Columbia University's prestigious Glenda Garvey Teaching Academy and has been recognized nationally for humanism in medicine by the Association of American Medical Colleges. He has developed several innovative education programs for stroke survivors and the general public, and under his leadership Harlem Hospital's Stroke Center received a special Proclamation of outstanding service from the City of New York in 2007. Dr. Williams has received numerous community service awards including the NAACP Community Service Award in 2008. He is on the National Spokesperson's Panel of the American Heart Association and the National Stroke Association.

Dr. Williams lives with his wife, Buki, daughter, Lola, and son, Tobi in New York, NY.